PLANT-BASED MEAL PREP

Fast and Easy Vegan Cookbook, 100 Tasty Plant-Based Recipes and Whole Foods, Including a 30-Day Time-Saving Meal Plan

By

KATE LIGHT

TABLE OF CONTENTS

Veganism. What is it and how can it improve my life? 7
The Alkaline Diet: Why it is Important for Optimal Health 12
Understanding Plant Micronutrients 14
Apple Buckwheat Pancakes With Coconut Caramel Apples.............16
Quick Vegan Breakfast Burritos 18
Chickpea Omelette 21
Gingerbread Waffles 23
Jelly-Filled Muffins 25
Toast with Refried Beans and Avocado 27
Sun-dried Tomato, Mushroom, and Spinach Tofu Quiche.............. 28
Vegan Breakfast Sandwich...30
Warm and Nutty Cinnamon Quinoa 31
Canal House Lentils 33
Hot Chocolate Banana-Nut Oatmeal... 34
Peanut Butter Banana Bread Granola 36
Broccoli and Quinoa Breakfast Patties 38
Salted Caramel Apple Breakfast Bars 40
Sweet Potato Breakfast Bowl 42
Grits Bowl with Avocado and Baked Tofu Strips 44
Greek Chickpeas on Toast.. 46
Breakfast Hash 48
Spinach Artichoke Quiche 50
Fried Tofu 52
Breakfast Turmeric Tofu 53
Deli-Style Vegan Cream Cheese Bowls.. 54
Cardamom and Peach Quinoa Porridge 55
Three-Grain Porridge... 56
Breakfast Fry-Up.. 57
Banana Bread 59
Easy Homemade Vegan Bread..61
Power Bread with Seeds... 63
Pear Pecan Bread 65
Naan Bread... 67
Pull-Apart Cinnamon Bread 69
Leftover Rice Bread...71
Biscuits 73
Vegan Cheese Jalapeño Biscuits.. 75

Rosemary Biscuits 77
Cream of Mushroom Soup 78
Beetroot and Lentil Tabbouleh 79
Creamy Cauliflower Horseradish Soup 80
No-Cook Chickpea Salad... 81
Silky Cauliflower Soup 82
Roasted Beets, Plum and Pecan Salad..............................83
Roasted Red Pepper Tomato Soup 84
Avocado Panzanella 85
Glowing Carrot Ginger Soup..86
Butter Bean, Cucumber and Radish Salad 88
Quinoa Black Bean Pumpkin Soup...................................89
Heirloom Tomato Salad...91
Healing Thai Butternut Squash Lentil Soup 92
Spiralized Zucchini and Carrot Salad...............................94
Winter Moroccan Sweet Potato Lentil Soup 95
Kale Power Salad with Lemon Tahini Dressing................ 97
Spring Vegetable Quinoa Minestrone 99
Cranberry Cilantro Quinoa Salad 101
Power Lentil Soup 103
Sweet Potato Salad.. 105
Roasted Vegetable Soup with Couscous.......................... 106
Fennel Asparagus Salad 108
Spicy Roasted Parsnip Soup 110
Farro Tabbouleh Salad...112
Minty Pea and Potato Soup 113
Italian Rice Noodles 114
Maple Glazed Tofu 115
Spaghetti with Kale 117
Lasagne (Vegan version)..119
Spanish Vegan Paella...122
Artichoke Mushroom Pizza...125
Tomato Chili Bean... 128
Sweet Potato Squash with Rice....................................... 130
Curry Beans 132
Fried Tofu and Edamame 134
Chili Spaghetti...136
French Stewed Vegetable (Ratatouille) 137
Spinach Puree and Sautéed Chickpea 138
Pasta with Beans 140

4

Vegan Enchiladas 141
Stuffed Peppers 144
Fried Pad Thai Rice Noodles 146
Juicy Sautéed Mushrooms and Corn... 148
Saffron Quinoa with Pistachios 150
Sautéed Cabbage 152
Fried Rice 153
Zucchini Balls with Pasta 155
Sloppy Joes..157
Mushroom Risotto 159
Milky Cauliflower Pasta 161
Potato Chips 163
Crackers with Edamame Hummus...165
Peanut Butter Jelly Apple Nachos 166
Fried Cinnamon Bananas 167
Maple Almond Popcorn 168
Turmeric Snack Balls 169
Herbed Fingerling Potatoes.. 170
Grilled Portobello Mushrooms 172
Jordanian Spiced Roasted Chickpeas...173
Spicy French Fries...174
Crusted Asparagus Spears 176
Buffalo Cauliflower Bites 177
Vegan 'Bacon' Strips...179
Fudgy Double Chocolate Apple Muffins...................................... 180
Salted Caramel Apple Bars 182
Lemon Cheesecake... 184
Lemon-Oatmeal Cookies.. 186
Coconut Chocolate Mousse 188
Chocolate Cupcakes 189
Lemon Poppy Seed Scones 191
Chocolate Chip Cookies 193
Brownies..195
No-Bake Lemon Tarts 197
Peanut Butter Caramel Rice Krispies 199
Guilt-Free Coconut Vanilla Macaroons 201
Gluten-Free Baked Chocolate Doughnuts...................................203
Peanut Butter Fudge 205
Tahini-Stuffed Dates 207
Dark Chocolate Truffles 209

Tahini Chocolate Banana Soft Serve 211
Thai Iced Tea...213
Chai Tea Lattes..215
Lemon Tulsi Tea...217
Peach Iced Tea.. 218
Rooibos and Pear Tea 219
Turmeric Tea..220
Green Tea with Grapefruit..221
Mint Tea 222
Sunshine Smoothie 223
Youthful Green Smoothie 224
Orange Cardamom Beet Smoothie 225
Peachy Mango Smoothie.. 226
Ginger and Spinach Green Smoothie 227
Oil-Free Balsamic Dressing 228
Creamy Red Pepper Coriander Sauce....................................... 229
Nacho Cheese Sauce.. 230
Ranch Dressing 231
Barbecue Tahini Sauce... 232
Whole Roasted Cauliflower with Tahini Sauce 233
Mushroom Pasta with Roasted Sunchokes 235
Berry Banana Smoothie Bowl.. 237
Sweet Potato Dhal 238
Simple Baked Sheet-Pan Ratatouille..240
Raw Apple Pie 243
Quick Mushroom and Lime Salad 244
Lentil Burger with Mustard Sauce... 246
30 Days Meal Plan 248
Conclusion.. 258
Disclaimer 260

VEGANISM. WHAT IS IT AND HOW CAN IT IMPROVE MY LIFE?

Veganism-a way of living that excludes the exploitation and cruel treatment of animals through food, clothing, or in any other form is currently becoming increasingly popular. In the past several years, lots of people decided to switch to veganism, and lots of vegan products appeared on store shelves.

The term "vegan" was first introduced back in 1944 by a group of vegetarians that separated from the Leicester Vegetarian Society in England to form the Vegan Society. The term was made from the first and last letters of word "vegetarian". In addition to not consuming meat they decided to stop consuming dairy, eggs, or any other products of animal origin as well.

Usually, people decide to go vegan due to one or several reasons. People might switch to veganism due to their ethical reasons, as they believe all live creatures have a right to live, be free, and fairly treated. That is why they are opposed to the idea of taking someone's life just for the sake of consuming or using any part of the animal. They also oppose the possible psychological and physical stress that animals might go through in modern farming practices.

Others choose veganism for health benefits that it provides. For example, plant-based diets may reduce the risk of heart disease, type 2 diabetes, cancer, premature death, Alzheimer's disease, various cancers, avoid side effects linked to the antibiotics and hormones used in modern animal agriculture, lower body weight and body mass index (BMI).

Another might prefer to go the other way because of the impact animal agriculture has on the environment, which is colossal. Animal agriculture makes up for up to 65% of global emissions of nitrous oxide, 35–40% of emissions of methane, and 9% of emissions of carbon dioxide, and these chemical compounds are the main drivers of climate change. On top of that, animal agriculture requires lots of water and can also lead to deforestation.

People that switched to veganism avoid consuming any animal products and products that have ingredients of animal origin.

- Meat, poultry, and products that contain any meat ingredients.

- Fish, seafood and products that contain any seafood ingredients.

- Dairy and products that contain any dairy

ingredients.

- Eggs and products that contain any egg ingredients.

- Bee products and products that contain any ingredients of that nature.

- Animal-based products and products that contain any animal-based ingredients.

If you are on a vegan diet, you do not have to eat only vegetables and fruits. Lots of usual dishes are already vegan or can be easily turned into vegan. And people that follow the vegan path have a wide variety of options to choose from to substitute animal products.

Seitan, tempeh, and tofu are versatile protein-rich options that can replace meat, poultry fish and eggs.

Peas, lentils, and beans have lots of nutrients and beneficial plant compounds.

Nuts and nut butter are a perfect choice in terms of fiber, iron, zinc, magnesium, selenium, and vitamin E.

Chia, flaxseeds, and hemp seeds contain protein and beneficial omega-3 fatty acids.

Calcium-fortified plant milk and yogurts help achieve the needed daily calcium intake.

Chlorella and spirulina have complete protein in them, while other varieties of algae have iodine.

Nutritional yeast has protein in it.

Whole grains, cereals, and pseudocereals can help with complex carbs, fiber, iron, B-vitamins and several minerals. To get as much protein as possible, choose spelled, teff, amaranth, and quinoa.

Ezekiel bread, tempeh, miso, natto, sauerkraut, pickles, kimchi, and kombucha have probiotics and vitamin K2. To improve mineral absorption do sprouting and fermenting before consumption.

Fruits and vegetables are great choices to increase nutrient intake.

Veganism also offers a variety of health benefits.

Vegan diet is rich in nutrients, and if you go from a Western diet to a vegan one, you will stop eating animal products and switch to plant-based foods you will start getting more fiber, antioxidants, beneficial plant compounds, potassium, magnesium, folate, and vitamins A, C, and E, which in result will improve your health. But this type of diet should be carefully planned to achieve that desired result.

Going vegan can also help with losing weight. Several

trusted studies show that vegan diets are more efficient when compared with other weight-loss diets. As a result vegans tend to be thinner and have lower body mass indexes (BMIs) than non-vegans.

A vegan diet may lower the risk of cancer and people on a vegan diet may have a 15% lower risk of getting cancer or die from it.

A vegan diet can be effective at reducing symptoms of arthritis such as pain, joint swelling, and morning stiffness.

It also improves kidney function and reduces the risk of poor performance.

It can also help with reducing the risk of developing Alzheimer's disease.

THE ALKALINE DIET: WHY IT IS IMPORTANT FOR OPTIMAL HEALTH

The alkaline diet, also known as the acid-alkaline diet or the alkaline ash diet is based around the idea of avoiding acid-forming foods and replacing them with alkaline foods. Its main idea is about altering the pH value, the measurement of acidity or alkalinity of the human body.

Metabolism, the process of converting the consumed food into energy, can be compared to a fire. It involves a chemical reaction that breaks down the consumed food into different components. And as with the fire, when food gets broken down, and ash residue in the form of metabolic waste is left behind. This leftover metabolic ash can be either acidic, neutral, or alkaline. Therefore, if the person is consuming food that is leaving the acidic metabolic ash, it can make blood acidic and, thus, directly affects the overall body's acidity and health as a result. And if the person eats food that leaves alkaline metabolic waste, then it will make blood alkaline. According to the theory about metabolic waste, acidic ash is what makes human health vulnerable to illness and disease, whereas alkaline metabolic waste improves health and makes it stronger.

Therefore, by eating alkaline food one should be able to make the body alkaline and improve health.

It is quite important to understand what pH is when talking about the alkaline diet, as pH is a tool to measure how acidic something is. The pH value ranges from 0 to 14, with acidic being between 0.0 to 6.9, neutral being 7.0, and alkaline ranging from 7.1 to 14.0. It should be mentioned that pH levels vary within the human body, with some parts being acidic and others being alkaline. pH level is an essential indicator of human health, and If it were to fall outside of the normal range, cells in the body would stop working and lead to death.

Food components that leave acidic ash include protein, phosphate, and sulfur, while alkaline components include calcium, magnesium, and potassium. Certain food groups are considered acidic, alkaline, or neutral. Acidic include meat, poultry, fish, dairy, eggs, grains, and alcohol. Neutral include natural fats, starches, and sugars. Alkaline include fruits, nuts, legumes, and vegetables.

UNDERSTANDING PLANT MICRONUTRIENTS

Macronutrients and micronutrients are molecules that the human body needs to survive, properly function and avoid getting ill. We need macros in large amounts, as they are the main nutrients for our body. There are 3 main macronutrients: carbohydrates, proteins, and fats. Micronutrients such as vitamins, minerals, and electrolytes are the other type of major nutrients that human body needs.

In comparison to macros, micros are required in much smaller amounts but play a vital role. The human body needs vitamins to produce energy, support of the immune system, blood clotting, etc, while minerals are needed for growth, bone health, fluid balance. To sum it up, micronutrients take part in nearly every process in the human body.

Micronutrients must be obtained from food sources since the human body cannot produce them on its own. And as the micronutrient content of food differs, a whole variety of food should be consumed to get an adequate intake of them to ensure optimal health. Micronutrients that include vitamins and minerals can be divided into four categories:

water-soluble vitamins, fat-soluble vitamins, macrominerals, and trace minerals.

Recent studies indicate that an adequate intake of micronutrients has great effects on human health. Research shows that sufficient consumption of vitamins A and C lower the risk of some cancers. Some vitamins may help prevent Alzheimer's disease. Research shows that low levels of selenium in blood heighten the risk of heart disease, and with the rise of selenium the risk of heart disease falls. Also, good levels of calcium decrease the risk of death from heart disease.

APPLE BUCKWHEAT PANCAKES WITH COCONUT CARAMEL APPLES

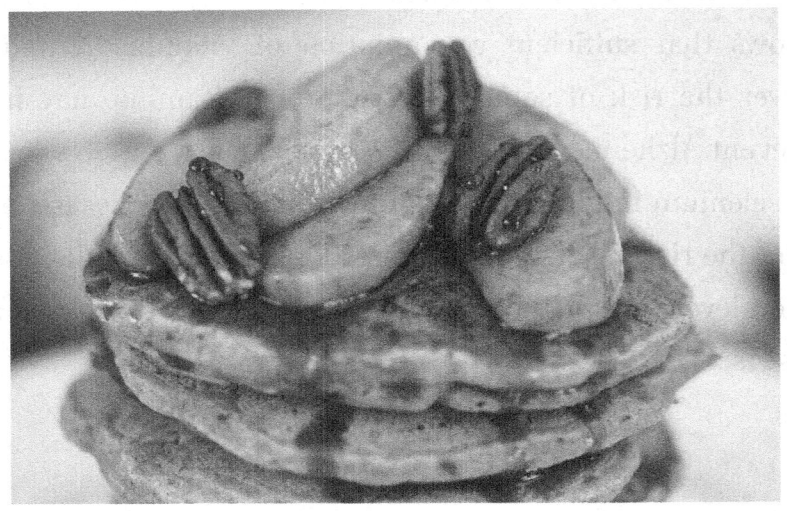

Cook Time: 60 minutes

Servings: 11 pancakes

Ingredients:

- 1 3/4 cups buckwheat flour
- 4 tablespoon coconut sugar
- 2 teaspoon baking powder
- 1/4 teaspoon vanilla powder
- 3 teaspoons cinnamon
- 1/4 teaspoon sea salt

- 2 tablespoons + 1 teaspoon coconut oil, melted
- 1 1/4 cups + 2 tablespoons almond milk
- 1 tablespoon flax seeds and 3 tablespoons water
- 1 cup apple chunks
- 1/4 teaspoon water
- 1 apple, peeled and cut into wedges

Instructions:

1. Prepare flax egg by mixing flax seeds and water. Let rest for 5 minutes. Add flour, baking powder, 2 tablespoons coconut sugar, vanilla powder, salt, and 2 teaspoons cinnamon to a bowl.
2. Mix flax egg with 1 1/4 cups almond milk and add to dry ingredients. Let pancake batter rest for 15 minutes. Add 2 tablespoon almond milk, chopped apple, and coconut oil.
3. Add few drops of coconut oil to a pan over medium-low heat and spread. Add 1/4 cup batter to it and cook for 3 minutes. Flip and cook for 2 minutes.
4. Add 1 teaspoon coconut oil, remaining coconut sugar, cinnamon and water in a pan. Mix and combine until smooth. Add apple wedges and cook until soft to make coconut caramel apples.
5. Serve caramel apples over pancakes.

QUICK VEGAN BREAKFAST BURRITOS

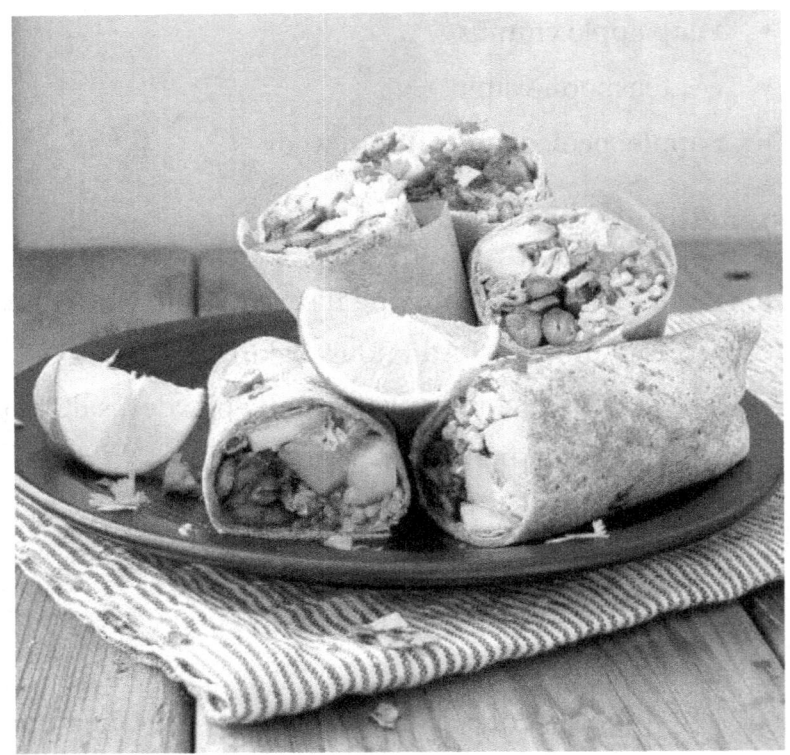

Cook Time: 30 minutes

Servings: 2 burritos

Ingredients:

- 1 1/2 cups water
- 3/4 cup white rice, rinsed and drained
- 1/2 + 1 lime juice

- 1/4 cup cilantro, chopped
- 1/2 teaspoon salt
- 1/2 red onion
- 4 red potatoes
- 2 tablespoons vegan butter
- 1/4 teaspoon black pepper
- 1 cup black beans, cooked
- 1/4 teaspoon chili, cumin and garlic powder
- 1/4 avocado
- 1 jalapeno, seeds removed and sliced
- 1 cup cabbage, sliced
- 2 vegan flour tortillas
- 1/4 cup salsa

Instructions:

1. Add rice, water, and 1/4 teaspoon salt to a pot and bring to boil. Reduce the heat to low, cover and cook for 20 minutes. Remove and set aside.

2. Wash and chop potatoes. Cut onion to 1/4" rings. Heat a skillet over medium heat. Add vegan butter and coat. Add potatoes to one side and onions to others. Season and cover and cook for 5 minutes on one side and 5 minutes on other. Remove and set aside.

3. Add beans to a pan placed over medium heat and season with garlic powder, cumin, and chili powder. Once bubbles form, reduce heat.

4. Mix avocado and 1 lime juice in a bowl. Add jalapeno and cabbage and mix. Season and set coleslaw aside. Add lime juice and cilantro to rice and toss.

5. Wrap tortillas in a towel and microwave for 30 seconds.

6. Add fillings in it, avocado and salsa. Roll into burritos, slice and serve.

CHICKPEA OMELETTE

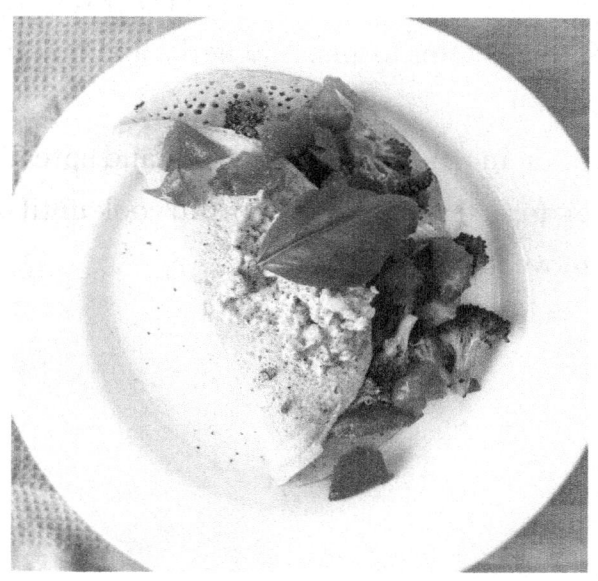

Cook Time: 5 minutes

Servings: 1

Ingredients:

- 3 tablespoons chickpea flour
- 8 tablespoons water
- 2 tablespoons oil
- 1 onion
- fresh herbs, to taste
- 1/2 teaspoon salt
- A pinch of black pepper

Instructions:

1. Combine flour with salt and pepper. Add water and mix until batter forms. Add herbs and onions in it. Mix well.
2. Heat oil in a pan. Add batter to it and spread evenly. Cook for a few minutes. Flip and cook until done.
3. Remove from heat and serve.

GINGERBREAD WAFFLES

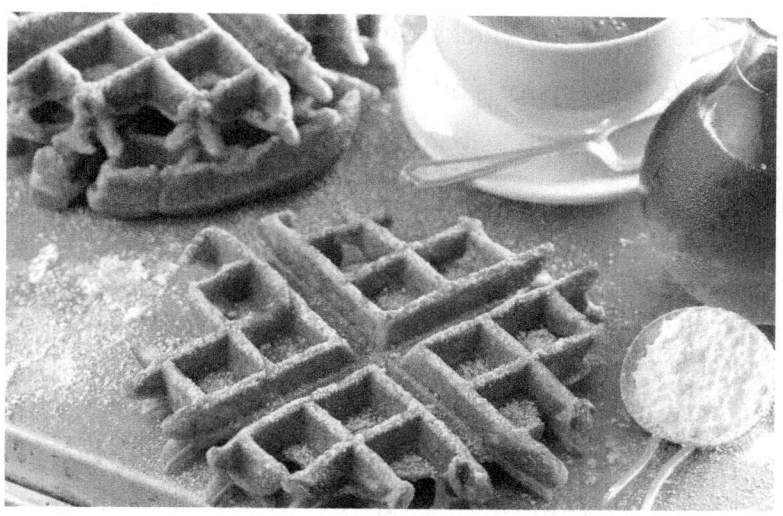

Cook Time: 15 minutes

Servings: 6

Ingredients:

- 1 tablespoon flax seeds
- 1 cup spelt flour
- 2 teaspoons baking powder
- 1 1/2 teaspoons cinnamon
- 4 tablespoons coconut sugar
- 2 teaspoons ginger
- 1/4 teaspoon salt
- 1/4 teaspoon baking soda

- 1 tablespoon apple cider vinegar
- 1 cup nondairy milk
- 2 tablespoons blackstrap molasses
- 1 1/2 tablespoons oil

Instructions:

1. Grease and preheat the waffle iron.
2. Mix flax seeds, flour, baking powder, cinnamon, coconut sugar, ginger, salt and baking soda in a bowl and stir well to combine.
3. Mixthe remaining ingredients in a separate bowl and stir well. Add wet ingredients to dry ones and mix until just combined.
4. Add the mixture to the waffle maker and cook as per the instructions. Serve and enjoy.

JELLY-FILLED MUFFINS

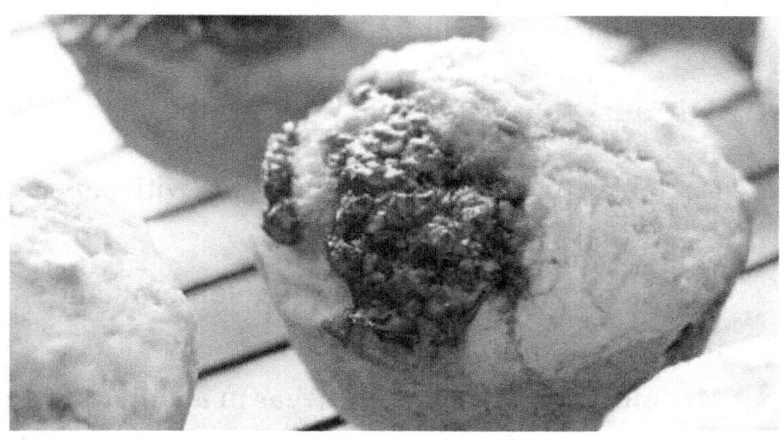

Cook Time: 25 minutes

Servings: 12

Ingredients:

- 3/4 teaspoon baking powder
- 1 1/2 cups all-purpose flour
- 1/2 teaspoon baking soda
- 1/2 teaspoon ground nutmeg
- 1 cup plain soy milk
- 1 teaspoon cider vinegar
- 3/4 cup and 2 tablespoons granulated sugar
- 2 tablespoons cornstarch
- 1/3 cup vegetable oil

- 2 teaspoons vanilla extract
- 1/3 cup strawberries jam
- 1/2 teaspoon fine salt

Instructions:

1. Heat oven to 350F. Line a muffin cup with paper liners and set aside.
2. Add baking soda, baking powder, flour, salt and nutmeg to a bowl. Make a well in the mixture.
3. Mix milk, cornstarch and vinegar in another bowl until cornstarch dissolves. Add to the well in the flour mixture. Add vanilla, oil and sugar and stir well.
4. Fill each muffin cup to three quarters. Create indentation by spreading batter slightly from middle to edges. Add 1 teaspoon jam into the well. Repeat with each.
5. Bake for 22 minutes. Let cool on a wire rack for 5 minutes. Remove, cool completely and serve.

TOAST WITH REFRIED BEANS AND AVOCADO

Cook Time: 5 minutes

Servings: 2

Ingredients:

- 1 cup vegan refried beans
- 2 sandwich bread slices
- 1 avocado, sliced
- Salt, to taste
- white onion, sliced

Instructions:

1. Toast the bread slices. Add avocado and beans on top.
2. Add onions and sprinkle salt over it.
3. Serve and enjoy!

SUN-DRIED TOMATO, MUSHROOM, AND SPINACH TOFU QUICHE

Cook Time: 50 minutes

Servings: 8

Ingredients:

- 1 cup almonds, grounded
- 1 tablespoon flax seeds + 3 tablespoon water, mixed
- 1 cup rolled oats, grounded
- 2 teaspoons dried oregano
- 1 teaspoon dried parsley
- 2 tablespoons olive oil
- 3 tablespoons water
- 1/2 teaspoon kosher salt
- 14 oz firm tofu
- 1 leek, sliced
- 3 garlic cloves, minced
- 3 cups cremini mushrooms, sliced
- 1/2 cup basil leaves, chopped
- 1/2 cup chives, chopped
- 1 cup baby spinach
- 1/3 cup oil-packed-sun dried tomatoes, chopped

- 2 tablespoons yeast
- 1 teaspoon sea salt

Instructions:

1. Preheat the oven to 350F and grease a tart pan. Drain water from the tofu completely.
2. Whisk flax and water in a bowl and let rest for 5 minutes: Mix oat flour, almond meal, parsley, 1 teaspoon oregano, and kosher salt in a bowl. Add 1 tablespoon oil and flax mixture. Stir until dough forms.
3. Add dough to the pan and spread evenly on the bottom. Poke some holes in it. Bake crust for 16 minutes, let cool, and increase oven temp to 375F.
4. Add tofu into a blender. Blend until smooth. Cook garlic and onion in a pan over medium heat for few minutes add mushrooms, season, and cook over medium-high for 12 minutes. Add herbs, yeast, spinach, tomatoes, salt, and oregano and combine well. Cook until spinach wilts.
5. Remove and mix in tofu. Add on top of the baked crust and smooth out. Bake for 37 minutes. Cool for 10 minutes and serve.

VEGAN BREAKFAST SANDWICH

Cook Time: 15 minutes

Servings: 1

Ingredients:

- 1 vegan sausage patty
- 1 English muffin
- 1 slice vegan cheese
- 1 teaspoon strawberry jam
- 1 teaspoon hot sauce
- 1/4 avocado, sliced

Instructions:

1. Toast the muffin well. Cook the patty in microwave for 1 minute. Add cheese on top and heat for 30 seconds.
2. Slice the toasted muffin and add spread the jam on top. Add patty and cheese. Add avocado.Serve and enjoy.

WARM AND NUTTY CINNAMON QUINOA

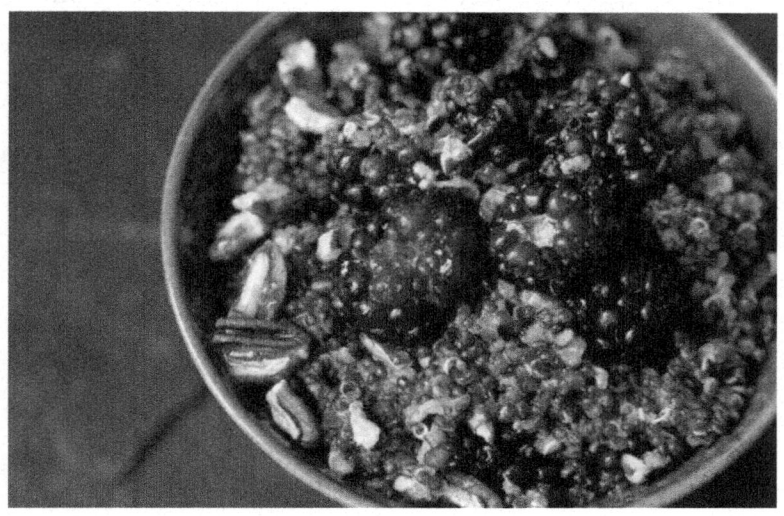

Cook Time: 20 minutes

Servings: 4

Ingredients:

- 1 cup of water
- 1 cup 1% low-fat milk, organic
- 2 cups blackberries
- 1 cup quinoa, organic
- 1/3 cup pecans, chopped and toasted
- 1/2 teaspoon cinnamon
- 4 teaspoons organic agave nectar

Instructions:

1. Mix water, quinoa, and milk in a pan. Bring to a boil over high heat. Reduce the heat, cover and cook for 15 minutes. Turn heat off and let sit for 5 minutes.
2. Add cinnamon and blackberries and transfer to 4 bowls. Add pecans. Add 1 teaspoon agave over each bowl.Serve and enjoy.

CANAL HOUSE LENTILS

Cook Time: 1 hour

Servings: 8

Ingredients:

- 1 leek, white and green parts, chopped
- 2 tablespoons olive oil
- 1 tablespoon tomato paste
- 1 garlic clove, sliced
- 1 cup green lentils
- 2 tablespoons soy sauce
- salt and pepper, to taste

Instructions:

1. Heat oil in a pan over medium heat. Add garlic, leek and tomato sauce and cook for 4 minutes.
2. Add 2 1/2 cups water and lentils. Bring to a boil. Reduce the heat, cover and cook for 55 minutes.
3. Remove from heat and let sit for 10 minutes. Add soy sauce and season to taste. Serve and enjoy.

HOT CHOCOLATE BANANA-NUT OATMEAL

Cook Time: 25 minutes

Servings: 4

Ingredients:

- 2 cups almond milk
- 1/4 teaspoon almond extract
- 2 ripe bananas (1 1/2 diced and 1 1/2 slices crosswise)
- 2 cups rolled oats
- 1/4 teaspoon vanilla extract
- 2 tablespoons cocoa powder
- 1/3 cup walnuts, toasted and chopped
- 2 tablespoons honey
- 2 tablespoons milk chocolate chips
- A pinch cinnamon

Instructions:

1. Add 1 3/4 cups water, almond milk, almond and vanilla extracts, diced bananas and pinch of salt to a pan and bring to a boil over high heat.
2. Add cocoa powder, oats and 1 tablespoon honey and reduce heat to medium. Cook for 7 minutes.

3. Transfer to 4 bowls and top with sliced bananas, honey, walnuts, chocolate chips and cinnamon.Serve and enjoy.

PEANUT BUTTER BANANA BREAD GRANOLA

Cook Time: 50 minutes

Servings: 6 cups

Ingredients:

- 3 cups rolled oats
- 1 cup salted peanuts
- 1 cup banana chips, crushed lightly
- 1/4 cup brown sugar
- 1/2 cup uncooked quinoa
- 1 teaspoon cinnamon
- 6 tablespoons butter, unsalted
- 1/3 cup peanut butter
- 1/4 cup pure honey
- 2 teaspoons vanilla extract
- 1/2 cup banana, mashed
- 1 teaspoon salt

Instructions:

1. Preheat the oven to 325F and line 2 rimmed baking sheets with parchment paper. Mix banana chips,

peanuts, oats, sugar, quinoa, cinnamon, and salt in a bowl.

2. Heat peanut butter, butter, and honey in a pan over medium-low heat for 4 minutes. Remove from heat and add vanilla and banana. Add to the oat mixture and mix well.

3. Spread granola onto the baking sheet — Bake for 27 minutes.

4. Cool on wire racks. Serve and enjoy.

BROCCOLI AND QUINOA BREAKFAST PATTIES

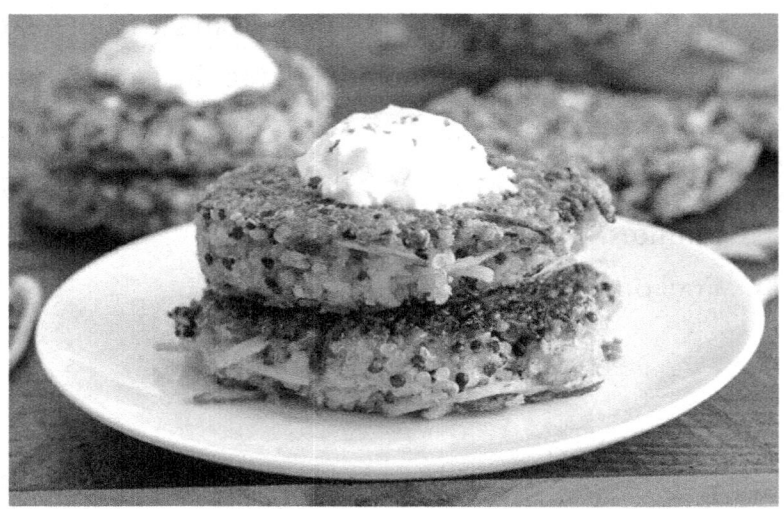

Cook Time: 25 minutes

Servings: 8

Ingredients:

- 2 cups vegetable broth
- 1 cup cooked quinoa
- 1 cup broccoli and carrots mixture, shredded
- 2 flax eggs
- 2 garlic cloves, minced
- 1/2 cup breadcrumbs, gluten-free
- 1 1/2 teaspoons garlic powder

- 2 teaspoons parsley
- 1 1/2 teaspoons onion powder
- 2 tablespoons coconut oil
- Salt and pepper, to taste

Instructions:

1. Rinse quinoa and add to a pan with vegetable broth. Once it boils, reduce the heat and cook for 15 minutes.
2. Add quinoa, flax eggs, shredded broccoli and carrots, garlic, parsley, breadcrumbs, 2 tablespoons oil, salt, and pepper to a bowl and mix well to combine.
3. Add little olive oil to the pan. Shape the mixture into balls and place them on the pan and flatten with the palm of your hand — Cook for 3 minutes per side.
4. Top with parsley and serve. Enjoy!

SALTED CARAMEL APPLE BREAKFAST BARS

Cook time: 30 minutes

Servings: 10 bars

Ingredients:

- 1 cup rolled oats
- 1 cup oat flour
- 1 teaspoon baking powder
- 2 apples, grated
- 3/4 cup medjol dates, pitted
- 3 tablespoon chia seeds
- 2/3 cup tahini
- 1 teaspoon vanilla extract
- 1/4 cup + 2 tablespoon plant milk
- 1/2 teaspoon salt

Instructions:

1. Preheat the oven to 350F. Mix baking powder, oats, oat flour and salt in a bowl. Mix well to combine. Add grated apples to a bowl.

2. Add tahini, dates, chia seeds, milk and vanilla extract to a blender and blend until smooth. Add the date

mixture and grated apples to the bowl with dry ingredients. Stir well.

3. Transfer the batter to a greased baking pan and bake for 30 minutes. Let cool for 10 minutes in the pan.

4. Remove, let cool completely, slice and serve. Enjoy!

SWEET POTATO BREAKFAST BOWL

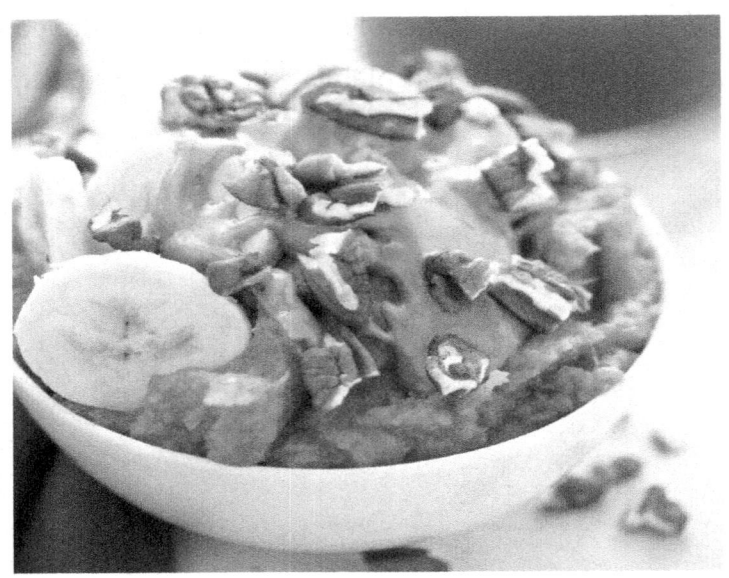

Cook Time: 1 hour 25 minutes

Servings: 2

Ingredients:

- 16 oz. sweet potato
- 2 tablespoons raisins
- 2 tablespoons almond butter
- 2 tablespoons chopped nuts
- Cinnamon, to taste

Instructions:

1. Preheat the oven to 375F. Poke potatoes with a fork and wrap in foil. Bake for 80 minutes. Let cool for 5 minutes and peel.
2. Mash the potatoes in a bowl, add cinnamon. Add to a bowl, top with raisins and nuts. Add almond butter. Serve and enjoy!

GRITS BOWL WITH AVOCADO AND BAKED TOFU STRIPS

Cook Time: 45 minutes

Servings: 4

Ingredients:

- 1/4 cup soy sauce
- 1 block tofu, sliced into strips
- 1/2 teaspoon onion powder
- 1 tablespoon olive oil
- 1 teaspoon turmeric
- 4 servings grits
- 1/2 cup nutritional yeast
- 1 avocado
- 2 tablespoons vegan margarine
- salt and pepper, to taste

Instructions:

1. Preheat the oven to 425F. Mix turmeric, soy sauce, olive oil, and onion powder in a bowl and toss with tofu strips. Let rest for 15 minutes.
2. Place the tofu strips on a lined baking sheet — Bake for 15 minutes on both sides.

3. Cook grits according to package directions and finish cooking when tofu is done. Add margarine and yeast and divide among 4 bowls.
4. Add 1/4 baked tofu strips, 1/4 avocado, and 1/4 tomatoes to each bowl. Season and serve.

GREEK CHICKPEAS ON TOAST

Cook Time: 35 minutes

Servings: 2

Ingredients:

- 3 shallots, diced
- 2 tablespoons olive oil
- 2 garlic cloves, diced
- 1/2 teaspoon cinnamon
- 1/2 teaspoon sweet paprika
- 1/4 teaspoon smoked paprika
- 1/2 teaspoon salt
- 2 large tomatoes, skinned
- 6 slices crusty bread, toasted
- 2 cups chickpeas, cooked
- A pinch of black pepper
- Kalamata olives, for serving

Instructions:

1. Heat oil on a pan over medium heat and fry shallots until done. Add garlic and cook until shallots are completely done, and garlic softens. Add all spices and cook for 2 minutes and mix well.

2. Roughly chop tomatoes and add to the pan with 2 tablespoons water. Cook on low medium until sauce thickens. Add cooked chickpeas and mix well. Season.
3. Add the mixture on top of the toasted bread and add olives.Serve and enjoy.

BREAKFAST HASH

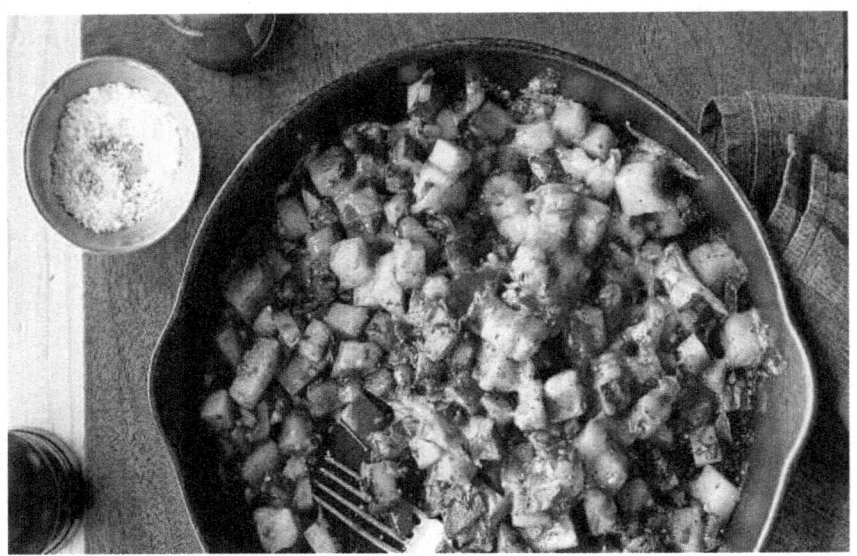

Cook Time: 1 hour

Servings: 6

Ingredients:

- 1 large sweet potato, peeled and diced
- 3 russet potatoes, peeled and diced
- 1 tablespoon garlic powder
- 1 tablespoon onion powder
- 1 teaspoon dried thyme
- 1/4 cup + 1 teaspoon olive oil
- 1 onion, diced

- 5 garlic cloves, minced
- Salt and pepper, to taste

Instructions:

1. Add potatoes, 1/4 cup olive oil, and spices to a bowl and mix well. Bake in a casserole dish at 450F for 50 minutes. Stir every 20 minutes.

2. Add olive oil in a skillet and cook onion and garlic for 8 minutes — season to taste.

3. Add potatoes to the onion/garlic mixture and mix well to combine — Cook for 1-2 minutes.

4. Serve and enjoy.

SPINACH ARTICHOKE QUICHE

Cook Time: 1 hour

Servings: 4

Ingredients:

- 2 large tortillas
- 1 tablespoon coconut oil
- 2 garlic cloves, minced
- 1/2 onion, chopped
- 2 cups spinach
- 1/2 cup nutritional yeast
- 14 oz. soft tofu
- 14 oz. can artichokes, drained and chopped
- 1 teaspoon Dijon mustard
- 1 teaspoon dried basil
- 1 lemon juice
- 1/2 teaspoon turmeric
- 1/4 teaspoon pepper
- 1/4 teaspoon salt

Instructions:

1. Preheat the oven to 350F and grease a pie dish with oil.

2. Cut tortillas in half and arrange on thepie dish —
   Bake for 15 minutes.
3. Heat oil in a pan. Add onion and cook for 5 minutes.
   Add garlic and cook for 2 minutes. Add spinach and
   cook until wilted. Remove.
4. Add spices, yeast, tofu, and lemon juice to a blender.
   Blend until smooth. Add onion mixture and
   artichokes to the blender and blend until mixed.
5. Transfer the mixture to the pie pan. Bake at 350F for
   45 minutes.Serve and enjoy.

FRIED TOFU

Cook Time: 20 minutes

Servings: 4

Ingredients:

- 1 block firm tofu, drained
- 1 tablespoon vegan butter
- Salt and pepper, to taste

Instructions:

1. Cut tofu into 4 thick slices. Cut off the corners of tofu to make a circle.
2. Melt butter in a pan over medium heat. Add tofu slices in a single layer. Fry until light brown on one side, flip and fry on the other side.
3. Remove and place on plates. Garnish and serve.

BREAKFAST TURMERIC TOFU

Cook Time: 15 minutes

Servings: 8

Ingredients:

- 2 packs (16 oz. each) firm tofu, packed in water
- 2 1/2 tablespoon nutritional yeast
- 1 1/4 teaspoon granulated garlic
- 2 tablespoons vegan margarine
- 1 1/4 teaspoon granulated onion
- 1/8 teaspoon turmeric
- 3/4 teaspoon sea salt
- 1/2 teaspoon black pepper

Instructions:

1. Drain water from the tofu. Add margarine to a skillet and turn the heat to medium. Add tofu and mix well.
2. Add onion, garlic, turmeric, salt and pepper to the pan. Mix and cook for 5 minutes on medium heat. Add yeast. Continue to cook until done.
3. Serve and enjoy!

DELI-STYLE VEGAN CREAM CHEESE BOWLS

Cook Time: 10 minutes

Servings: 2 cups

Ingredients:

- 8 1/2 oz. firm silken tofu
- 1 tablespoon ume plum vinegar
- 1 tablespoon white wine vinegar
- 1/2 teaspoon garlic powder
- 2 tablespoons white onion, minced
- 2 tablespoons red bell pepper, seeded and minced
- 2 tablespoons carrot, minced
- 2 tablespoons cucumber, minced
- 1 teaspoon sea salt

Instructions:

1. Drain water from tofu. Mix vinegars, tofu, salt and garlic powder in a blender and blend until smooth.
2. Transfer to a bowl and add the veggies. Serve and enjoy.

CARDAMOM AND PEACH QUINOA PORRIDGE

Cook Time: 20 minutes

Servings: 2

Ingredients:

- 1/3 cup porridge oats
- 1/2 cup quinoa
- 4 cardamom pods
- 2 peaches, cut into slices
- 1 teaspoon maple syrup
- 8 1/2 oz. almond milk

Instructions:

1. Add cardamom, oats and quinoa to a pan with 9 oz. water and 3 1/2 oz. milk. Bring to a boil and cook for 15 minutes.
2. Add the remaining milk and cook for 5 minutes. Remove the cardamom pods, divide the mixture among bowls and add peaches and maple syrup.Serve and enjoy.

THREE-GRAIN PORRIDGE

Cook Time: 10 minutes

Servings: 10-12

Ingredients:

- 3 1/2 cups oatmeal
- 3 1/2 cups barley flakes
- 3 1/2 cups spelled flakes
- agave nectar

Instructions:

1. Toast oatmeal, barley, and spelled flakes in a pan one by one for 5 minutes. Let cool and combine. Store in the airtight container in a dark dry place.
2. Add 2 oz of this mixture to 1 3/4 cups water in a pan and cook for 5 minutes (for 1 portion). Top with agave and serve.

BREAKFAST FRY-UP

Cook Time: 30 minutes

Servings: 4

Ingredients:

- 1 large potato, unpeeled
- 14 cherry potatoes
- 12 1/2 oz. silken tofu
- 1 1/2 tablespoons peanut butter
- 2 teaspoons maple syrup
- 1 teaspoon soy sauce
- 1 Portobello mushroom, sliced
- 1/4 teaspoon smoked paprika
- 2 tablespoons nutritional yeast
- 1 garlic clove, crushed
- 1/2 teaspoon turmeric
- 4 vegan sausages
- 1 cup black beans
- Sunflower oil

Instructions:

1. Cook whole potato in a pot of water, boil for 10 minutes and drain and cool. Peel and grate. Mix with

peanut butter and season to taste. Refrigerate before serving.

2. Heat the oven to 400 F. Add cherry tomatoes to a baking tray, add 2 teaspoon sunflower oil, season and bake for 30 minutes. Cook sausages and beans according to the package directions.

3. Mix soy sauce, maple syrup and 1/4 teaspoon paprika in a bowl. Add mushrooms and toss to coat.

4. Add 2 teaspoon oil to a pan and heat to medium-high. Fry mushroom until start to golden. Transfer to a plate.

5. Add 1 tablespoon oil to a pan and add spoonfuls of potato mixture. Cook for 4 minutes per side and drain add tofu to the pan and add the remaining ingredients and season to taste.

6. Fry tofu for 4 minutes. Divide everything among plates and serve. Enjoy!

BANANA BREAD

Cook Time: 50 minutes

Servings: 8

Ingredients:

- 1 1/3 cups banana, mashed
- 1/3 cup almond milk
- 2 tablespoons ground flaxseeds
- 1/3 cup coconut oil, melted
- 2 teaspoons vanilla extract
- 2 tablespoons maple syrup
- 1/2 cup rolled oats
- 1/4 cup + 2 tablespoons coconut sugar
- 1 teaspoon baking soda
- 1/2 teaspoon baking powder
- 1 1/2 cups whole-grain spelt flour
- 1/2 teaspoon salt

Instructions:

1. Preheat the oven to 350F and grease a loaf pan with cooking spray.

2. Add mashed banana to a bowl and add milk, ground flax, melted oil, vanilla, and maple syrup to it. Combine well.

3. Add sugar, oats, baking soda, baking powder, salt, and flour to the bowl and stir to combine. Transfer the dough to the pan and spread evenly.

4. Bake for 55 minutes. Place on a cooling rack for 30 minutes.Remove from the loaf pan and let cool completely.

5. Slice and serve. Enjoy!

EASY HOMEMADE VEGAN BREAD

Cook Time: 40 minutes

Servings: 10

Ingredients:

- 1 1/4 cup warm water
- 4 teaspoon active yeast
- 1 teaspoon sugar
- 2 1/2 cup all-purpose flour, gluten-free
- 1 tablespoon baking powder
- 1 cup oat flour
- 4 teaspoon xanthan gum
- 1 tablespoon apple cider vinegar
- 2 tablespoon olive oil
- 1 1/2 teaspoon salt

Instructions:

1. Add yeast to 1/4 cup warm water and mix with 1 teaspoon sugar. Let sit for 5 minutes.
2. Mix all dry ingredients in a separate bowl. Mix yeast mixture with dry ingredients and add 1/2 cup water,

vinegar, and oil. Mix until dough forms. Knead the dough for 5 minutes. Knead and shape into a loaf.

3. Transfer to a parchment-lined loaf pan and spread. Cover with a cotton towel and place in a warm place. Let sit for 80 minutes.

4. Score top of the loaf with knife, dust with flour and place in the oven and bake for 40 minutes at 350F. Brush with 1 tablespoon vegan butter 10 minutes before the end of cooking time.

5. Let cool for 15 minutes, slice and serve. Enjoy!

POWER BREAD WITH SEEDS

Cook Time: 50 minutes

Servings: 8

Ingredients:

- 2 tablespoons psyllium husk
- 1 1/2 cups water
- 1/2 cup raw almonds
- 1/3 cup flax seeds
- 1/2 cup sunflower seeds
- 1/3 cup sesame seeds, hulled
- 1/3 cup pumpkin seeds
- 1/2 cup dried currants
- 1 1/2 cups rolled oats
- 3 tablespoons coconut oil, melted
- 3/4 teaspoons sea salt

Instructions:

1. Add 1 1/2 cups water to a bowl and add psyllium husk and let sit for 10 minutes.
2. Add flax seeds, almonds, sunflower seeds, pumpkin seeds and sesame seeds to a blender. Blend to chop and add to psyllium husk after 10 minutes.

3. Add currants, salt, coconut oil and rolled oats to psyllium mixture. Mix well. Oil two baking tins and add seed mixture to it. Let sit for 1 hour and preheat oven to 350F.
4. Bake for 50 minutes. Let cool and serve. Enjoy!

PEAR PECAN BREAD

Cook Time: 50 minutes

Servings: 8

Ingredients:

- 1/4 cup tapioca starch
- 3/4 cup pecan meal
- 1/4 cup potato starch
- 2 teaspoons baking powder
- 1/4 cup coconut flour
- 1/4 teaspoon baking soda
- 1/2 teaspoon xanthan gum
- 1/2 teaspoon stevia powder
- 1/2 teaspoon ground nutmeg
- 3/4 cup pear, peeled and pureed
- 2 tablespoons plant-based milk
- 1 teaspoon vanilla

Instructions:

1. Preheat the oven to 350F. Chop pecans in a blender until crumbled. Mix pecans with the remaining dry ingredients in a bowl.

2. Add pear, vanilla, and milk to the bowl. Mix well to combine.
3. Transfer the batter to a greased loaf pan. Bake for 50 minutes. Let cool and serve. Enjoy!

NAAN BREAD

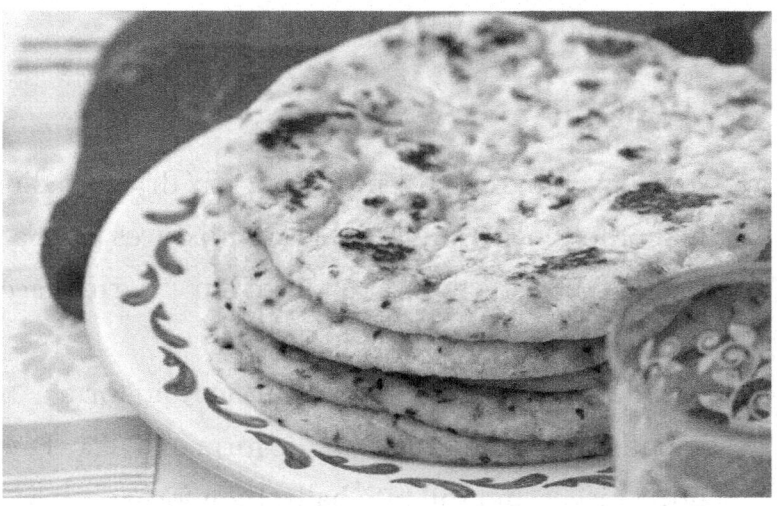

Cook Time: 10 minutes

Servings: 8

Ingredients:

- 1 cup non-dairy milk
- 1 tablespoon olive oil
- 1/2 cup non-dairy yogurt
- 1/4 cup cornstarch
- 2 cups all-purpose flour, gluten-free
- 1 teaspoon psyllium husk powder
- 1 teaspoon active dry yeast
- 1 teaspoon sugar

- 1/2 teaspoon salt
- 1/4 cup olive oil
- 1 tablespoon sesame seeds

Instructions:

1. Mix all wet ingredients in a bowl. Mix dry ingredients in another bowl. Combinethe two mixtures form a dough. Cover the bowl and place it in a warm place for 5 hours to let the dough rise.

2. Kneadthe dough on a floured surface and form a smooth ball and flatten it to the form of a disc. Divide into 8 pieces and roll into balls, then form discs.Brush with oil and sprinkle sesame seeds on top.

3. Set the oven to broil and grease a metal baking sheet. Place naan on it. Bake each side for 1 1/2 minutes. Flip when large bubbles form.Serve and enjoy.

PULL-APART CINNAMON BREAD

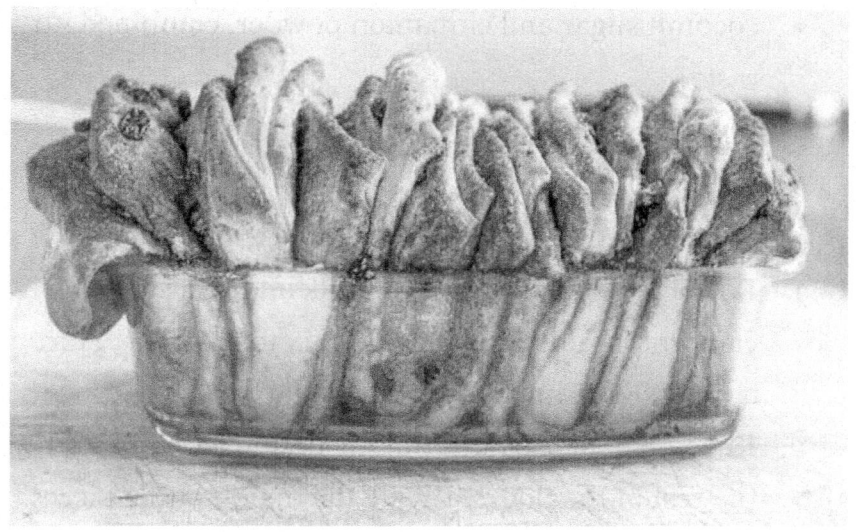

Cook Time: 35 minutes

Servings: 8

Ingredients:

- 2 cups non-dairy milk
- 5 3/4 tablespoons fresh yeast
- 1 flax egg
- 3/4 cup + 1 1/2 tablespoons coconut sugar
- 2 tablespoons cardamom
- 7 tablespoons walnut oil
- 7 tablespoons vegan butter

- 4 cups white flour, gluten-free
- 14 oz. mixture tapioca, almond, teff, and lupin flour
- coconut sugar and cinnamon powder, combined, to taste
- 1 teaspoon of sea salt

Instructions:

1. Dissolve yeast in lukewarm milk and add sugars, cardamom, salt, and flax and mix to combine. Start adding flours and stir well.
2. Knead half of the butter in the dough with oil. Add the rest of the flours. Divide the dough into 2 pieces and roll into a flat rectangle. Melt the remaining butter and brush the dough with it.Coat with vanilla, cinnamon, and sugar.
3. Slice rectangle into strips. Stack them on each other and cut into equal pieces. Place into the bread pan. Place bread in a warm place and let rise.
4. Brush with the egg mixture and bake at 350F for 35 minutes.Serve and enjoy.

LEFTOVER RICE BREAD

Cook Time: 45 minutes

Servings: 8

Ingredients:

- 3 cups flour
- 4 teaspoons oil
- 1 cup of rice, cooked
- 3/4 cup warm water
- 1 tablespoon sugar
- 2 1/4 teaspoons instant dry yeast
- 3/4 teaspoon salt

Instructions:

1. Add flour, 3 teaspoon oil, and salt to a bowl and mix well. Add sugar, yeast, and water to another bowl and let sit for 10 minutes. Add rice and mix well.
2. Add wet ingredients to the flour mix and knead for 7 minutes to form a dough. Add water while kneading as needed.
3. Transfer the dough to a greased bowl and evenly coat with oil. Cover and place in a warm place for 1 hour to rise.

4. Grease a loaf pan. Knead the butter again and add to the loaf pan.
5. Bake in a preheated oven for 45 minutes at 360F. Cool completely and slice. Serve and enjoy.

BISCUITS

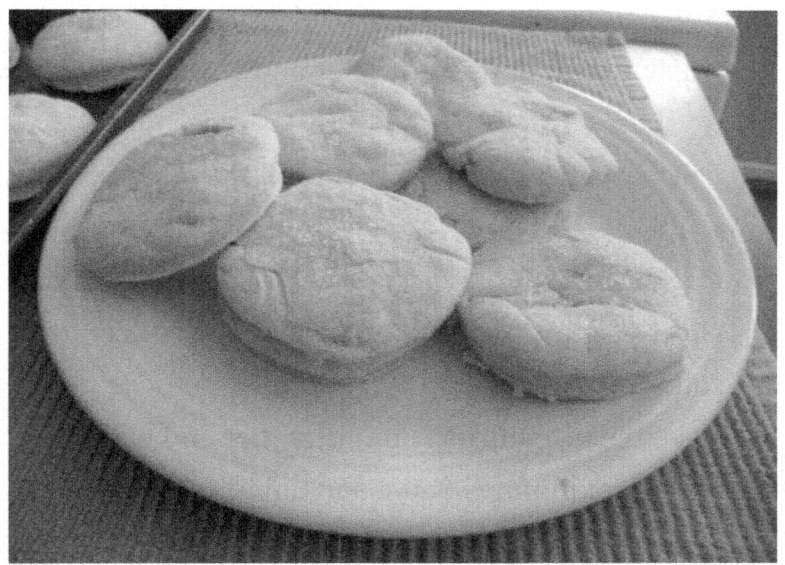

Cook Time: 25 minutes

Servings: 8

Ingredients:

- 2 cups white spelt flour
- 1/3 cup coconut oil
- 1 tablespoon baking powder
- 3/4 cup hot water
- 1 teaspoon salt

Instructions:

1. Preheat the oven to 375F and grease a baking sheet with coconut oil.
2. Add baking powder, flour, and salt to a bowl and whisk to combine. Add water and coconut oil. Stir until mixed well.
3. Dust a surface with flour and roll the dough outuntil 1" thick.
4. Cut the dough into biscuits and place on a baking sheet 1" apart. Brush each with oil and season with salt.
5. Bake the biscuits for 4 minutes, flip and bake for another 4 minutes.Serve and enjoy.

VEGAN CHEESE JALAPEÑO BISCUITS

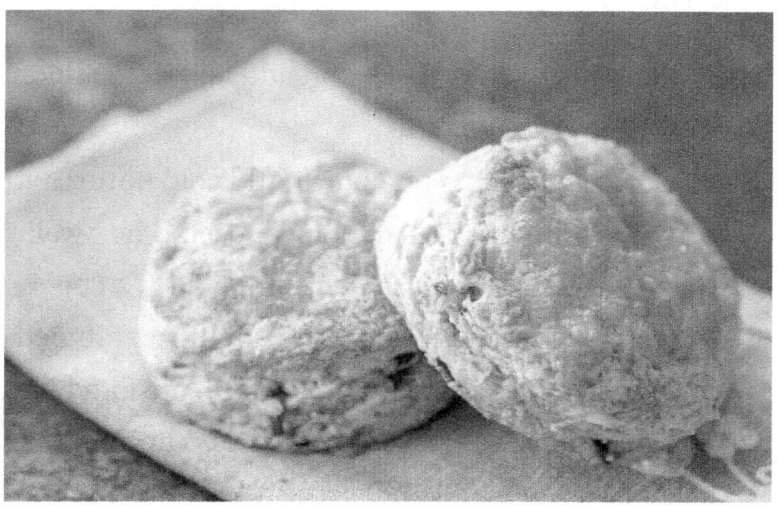

Cook Time: 30 minutes

Servings: 10 biscuits

Ingredients:

- 1 cup almond milk, unsweetened
- 2 cups all-purpose flour, bleached
- 1 tablespoon lemon juice
- 3 tablespoons nutritional yeast
- 1/2 teaspoon baking soda
- 1 tablespoon baking powder
- 4 tablespoons vegan butter, unsalted

- 1/4 cup jalapeno, seeds removed and diced
- 3/4 teaspoon sea salt

Instructions:

1. Preheat the oven to 450F and add lemon to almond milk.
2. Mix dry ingredients in a bowl. Add cold butter and combine with hands. Add jalapenos and mix well.
3. Make a well in dry ingredients and add 1/4 cup almond milk mixture. Stir until slightly combined.
4. Place the dough on a floured surface, dust and knead for 5 minutes. Roll out into a 1" disc. Cut into biscuits.
5. Place the biscuits on the baking sheet in 2 rows. Dust the top with butter. Bake for 15 minutes.Let cool and serve. Enjoy!

ROSEMARY BISCUITS

Cook Time: 35 minutes

Servings: 8 biscuits

Ingredients:

- 2 teaspoons baking powder
- 2 cups flour
- 4 tablespoons cold vegan butter
- 1 cup almond milk
- 1 tablespoon rosemary, chopped
- 1 teaspoon salt

Instructions:

1. Preheat the oven to 425F. Mix baking powder, flour, salt and rosemary in a bowl. Grate butter into this mixture. Mix in the liquid and stir until dough forms.

2. Place the mixture on a floured surface and knead a few times. Roll dough to 1" thickness. Cut out the biscuits from it.

3. Place on a baking sheet and bake for 15 minutes.Serve.

CREAM OF MUSHROOM SOUP

Cook Time: 20 minutes

Servings: 6

Ingredients:

- 16 oz. butter mushrooms, sliced
- 2 tablespoons vegan butter
- 1 yellow onion, chopped
- 3 garlic cloves, minced
- 4 cups vegetable broth
- 1/4 cup all-purpose flour
- 1 teaspoon dried thyme leaves
- 1 1/2 cups full-fat coconut milk
- 1/4 teaspoon nutmeg
- 1/2 teaspoon salt and pepper

Instructions:

1. Melt vegan butter in a pot over medium-high heat. Add onion, mushrooms, and garlic and cook until mushrooms are softened.
2. Add flour, stir and cook for 1 minute.
3. Add coconut milk, vegetable broth, thyme, nutmeg, salt, and pepper. Bring to a simmer and cook for 5 minutes more. Serve and enjoy.

BEETROOT AND LENTIL TABBOULEH

Cook Time: 15 minutes

Servings: 4

Ingredients:

- 1lb radishes
- 1 small pack mint
- 1 small pack chives
- 1 red apple, cored, quartered and sliced
- 2 beetroots, peeled and quartered
- 1 teaspoon ground cumin
- 4 tablespoons olive oil
- 2 lemons, juiced
- 1 1/2 cups cooked quinoa
- 2 cups chickpeas, drained and rinsed
- 2 cups green lentils, drained

Instructions:

1. Add radishes, herbs and beetroot to a blender and blend into chopped pieces.
2. Transfer to a bowl. Add the remaining ingredients and toss well to combine.
3. Season to taste. Serve and enjoy.

CREAMY CAULIFLOWER HORSERADISH SOUP

Cook Time: 20 minutes

Servings: 4

Ingredients:

- 2 potatoes, chopped
- 1 cauliflower, chopped
- 1 onion, chopped
- 3 cups vegetable broth
- 4 teaspoons horseradish sauce
- 1 teaspoon dried thyme
- 1 cup non-dairy milk
- Salt and pepper, to taste

Instructions:

1. Add potatoes, cauliflower, garlic, onion and vegetable broth, thyme and milk to a pan.
2. Bring to a boil, reduce the heat to low and simmer and cook for 15 minutes.
3. Transfer to a blender and blend until smooth. Return to the pan and add horseradish to taste. Season and serve. Enjoy!

NO-COOK CHICKPEA SALAD

Cook Time: 10 minutes

Servings: 6

Ingredients:

- 1 red onion, sliced
- 2 large tomatoes, chopped
- 1 lemon juice
- 2 tablespoons olive oil
- 2 tablespoons harissa
- 2 cups chickpeas, drained and rinsed
- 1 small pack parsley, chopped
- 1 small pack coriander, chopped

Instructions:

1. Add all ingredients to a large bowl. Toss well to combine.
2. Mash a little with a fork. Serve and enjoy.

SILKY CAULIFLOWER SOUP

Cook Time: 30 minutes

Servings: 2

Ingredients:

- 1 small head cauliflower
- 2 garlic cloves, minced
- 1 tablespoon olive oil
- 2 thyme sprigs
- 1/2 cup coconut milk
- 1 1/2 cups vegetable stock
- 4 tablespoons pomegranate seeds
- salt and pepper, to taste

Instructions:

1. Chop the cauliflower head into florets.
2. Cook garlic in olive oil in a skillet for 2 minutes. Add thyme sprigs, vegetable stock, and cauliflower. Bring to a boil, cover, reduce the heat and cook for 20 minutes.
3. Remove thyme and blend the soup until smooth. Add coconut milk and season with salt and pepper.Serve and enjoy.

ROASTED BEETS, PLUM AND PECAN SALAD

Cook Time: 30 minutes

Servings: 4

Ingredients:

- 4 ripe plums, cut into wedges
- 4 beetroots, peeled, ends trimmed and spiralized
- 2 1/2 tablespoons olive oil
- 1/2 tablespoon red wine vinegar
- 1/2 tablespoon pomegranate molasses
- 1/2 cup pecans, toasted and chopped
- 1 small pack mint leaves

Instructions:

1. Heat the oven to 400F.
2. Toss spiralized beetroot in 1 tablespoon olive oil and season well, spread out in one layer on a baking dish. Roast for 15 minutes.
3. Mix red wine vinegar, molasses and remaining olive oil in a bowl and season to taste.
4. Add the rest of the ingredients to a bowl and add beetroot. Add the dressing to it. Toss well to coat. Serve and enjoy.

ROASTED RED PEPPER TOMATO SOUP

Cook Time: 50 minutes

Servings: 4

Ingredients:

- 16 oz. tomatoes, sliced in half
- 1 1/4 lbs red bell peppers, seeded and sliced in quarters
- 2 carrots, chopped
- 1/2 red onion, cut into wedges
- 2 cups vegetable broth
- 1 tablespoon basil leaves, chopped
- 1/2 teaspoon salt

Instructions:

1. Preheat the oven to 450F and line a baking sheet with foil or parchment paper.
2. Spread veggies in a layer on the baking sheet and roast for 40 minutes and remove from oven. Let cool.
3. Peel the skin off peppers. Add veggies to a blender. Add the vegetable broth, a pinch of salt, and basil. Blend until smooth.
4. Add back to the pot, heat, and serve.

AVOCADO PANZANELLA

Cook Time: 20 minutes

Servings: 4

Ingredients:

- 1 3/4 lbs mixed ripe tomatoes
- 1 1/2 tablespoon capers, drained and rinsed
- 1 garlic clove, crushed
- 1 avocado, stoned, peeled and chopped
- 4 tablespoons olive oil
- 1 red onion, sliced
- 2 tablespoons red wine vinegar
- Ciabatta
- Basil leaves

Instructions:

1. Chop the tomatoes and add them to a bowl. Season then add capers, onion, garlic, and avocado and mix well. Let rest for 10 minutes.
2. Slice ciabatta into thick pieces and add to a bowl. Add half ofthe olive oil, half of vinegar and season. Add over the tomatoes.
3. Add basil leaves and the remaining olive oil and vinegar. Stir and serve. Enjoy.

GLOWING CARROT GINGER SOUP

Cook Time: 50 minutes

Servings: 6 cups

Ingredients:

- 1 lb. carrots, peeled and chopped
- 1 onion, diced
- 1 apple, diced
- 3 tablespoons avocado oil
- 3 cups vegetable broth
- 1 teaspoon garlic, minced
- 1 cup vanilla almond milk, unsweetened
- 1 tablespoon ginger, minced
- 1/2 teaspoon turmeric
- Salt and pepper, to taste

Instructions:

1. Preheat the oven to 425F. Spread onion, chopped carrots, and apple on a baking sheet.
2. Add oil and season with salt and pepper. Toss to combine. Roast for 15 minutes, toss and roast for 15 more minutes. Remove and set aside.

3. Add garlic, milk, broth, ginger, turmeric, and veggies to a blender. Blend until smooth. Season well.
4. Add to a pot, heat and serve. Enjoy!

BUTTER BEAN, CUCUMBER AND RADISH SALAD

Cook Time: 15 minutes

Servings: 3

Ingredients:

- 4 cups butter beans, drained and rinsed
- 2 garlic cloves, crushed
- 1 tablespoon olive oil
- 1/2 lemon juice and zest
- 1/2 cucumber, seeds removed and sliced into half-moons
- 1/2 lb. radish, trimmed and sliced
- 1 small bunch mint, chopped
- 1 small bunch parsley, chopped

Instructions:

1. Add parsley, lemon juice, and zest, garlic, mint and olive oil to a bowl to make the dressing.
2. Add radishes, butter beans, and cucumber to the bowl and mix well.Serve and enjoy.

QUINOA BLACK BEAN PUMPKIN SOUP

Cook Time: 35 minutes

Servings: 4

Ingredients:

- 20 oz. can black beans, rinsed and drained
- 1 tablespoon olive oil
- 5 garlic cloves, diced
- 1 onion, diced
- 1 red chili pepper, diced
- 3 cups pumpkin cubes
- 1/2 teaspoon dried oregano
- 1 teaspoon ground cumin
- 1/2 teaspoon red pepper flakes, crushed
- 1/2 cup quinoa
- 5 cups vegetable broth
- 2 bay leaves
- 1 lime, cut into wedges
- 1 avocado, cubed
- Handful cilantro, diced

Instructions:

1. Heat oil in a pan over medium heat. Add onion and cook for a few minutes. Add red chili pepper and garlic and cook until fragrant. Add spices and pumpkin and cook for 2 minutes.
2. Add quinoa and 2 cups vegetable broth. Bring to a boil, cook for 5 minutes and add the rest of vegetable broth. Bring to a boil.
3. Add bay leaves and beans. Bring to a boil, reduce the heat and cook for 10 minutes.
4. Garnish with lime juice, cilantro, and avocado. Serve and enjoy.

HEIRLOOM TOMATO SALAD

Cook Time: 15 minutes

Servings: 6

Ingredients:

- 2 tablespoons vinegar
- 1/4 cup olive oil
- 16 oz. cherry tomatoes halved
- 1 teaspoon honey
- 2 tablespoons chives, chopped
- 1 lb heirloom tomatoes, some sliced and some cut into wedges
- basil leaves
- salt and pepper, to taste

Instructions:

1. Mix oil, honey, vinegar, and 1/2 teaspoon salt and pepper in a bowl. Add chives and cherry tomatoes and toss to coat.
2. Add heirloom tomatoes to a plate and add 1/4 teaspoon salt and pepper. Add cherry tomato mixture.
3. Top with basil leaves and chives.Serve and enjoy.

HEALING THAI BUTTERNUT SQUASH LENTIL SOUP

Cook Time: 50 minutes

Servings: 4

Ingredients:

- 1 large carrot, diced
- 1/2 tablespoon olive oil
- 3 garlic cloves, minced
- 1 yellow onion, diced
- 1 tablespoon ginger, grated
- 1 tablespoon yellow curry powder
- 2 lbs butternut squash, peeled and cubed
- 1 tablespoon turmeric, grated
- 3 cups vegetarian broth, low sodium
- 15 oz. can light coconut milk
- 1 cup green lentils, rinsed and sorted
- 3 cups spinach
- 2 tablespoons creamy peanut butter
- Salt, pepper, to taste

Instructions:

1. Add coconut oil to a pot and heat over medium-high. Add ginger, garlic, and onion and cook for 5 minutes.
2. Add butternut squash cubes and carrot and cook for few minutes. Add turmeric and curry powder. Cook for 30 seconds and add coconut milk, lentils, vegetarian broth, and peanut butter — season to taste.
3. Bring to a boil, cover, reduce the heat to low and cook for 20 minutes more.
4. Transfer half of the soup to a blender. Blend slowly then increase speed. Add puree back to the pot with the remaining soup and mix well. Add spinach and cook until wilted.Season to taste, serve and enjoy.

SPIRALIZED ZUCCHINI AND CARROT SALAD

Cook Time: 25 minutes

Servings: 6

Ingredients:

- 2 tablespoons peanut oil, toasted
- 1/4 cup lime juice
- 2 tablespoons brown sugar
- 1 tablespoon soy sauce
- 1 1/2 teaspoons ginger, grated
- 1 large carrot, thinly spiralized
- 2 large zucchini, spiralized
- 2 scallions, sliced
- 1 red chile, sliced
- 1/2 cup peanuts, chopped and roasted
- 1/3 cup cilantro, chopped

Instructions:

1. Mix peanut oil, lime juice, ginger, soy sauce and brown sugar in a bowl.
2. Add carrots, zucchini, red chili and scallions. Toss well to coat.
3. Add cilantro and peanuts. Serve and enjoy.

WINTER MOROCCAN SWEET POTATO LENTIL SOUP

Cook Time: 6 hours 15 minutes

Servings: 8

Ingredients:

- 1 cup carrots, chopped
- 1 lb. sweet potatoes, peeled and cubed into pieces
- 1 cup onions, chopped
- 1 red bell pepper, diced
- 1 cup celery, chopped
- 6 garlic cloves, minced
- 1 1/2 teaspoon coriander and cumin powder each
- 1 1/2 cups green lentils, rinsed and picked over
- 1 teaspoon curry powder
- 1/8 teaspoon ground nutmeg
- 1/2 teaspoon smoked paprika
- 1/2 teaspoon ground cinnamon
- 1/2 teaspoon turmeric
- 7 cups vegetable broth, low sodium
- 2 1/2 cups baby spinach, chopped
- 1/4 cup lemon juice

Instructions:

1. Add carrots, sweet potatoes, celery, onions, red bell pepper, garlic, lentils, spices, and 6 cups broth to a slow cooker. Cover and cook for 5 hours on high. Lentils should be done.

2. Add half of the soup to a blender with 1/2 cup broth and blend until smooth. Add back to the slow cooker.

3. Add lemon juice and baby spinach. Cover, turn off the cooker and let rest for 30 minutes.

4. Season with curry powder, salt, and pepper. Serve and enjoy.

KALE POWER SALAD WITH LEMON TAHINI DRESSING

Cook Time: 40 minutes

Servings: 6

Ingredients:

- 2 sweet potatoes, peeled and diced
- 1 bunch curly kale, stems removed and chopped
- 1 tablespoon + 2 teaspoons olive oil
- 1 1/2 large lemon, juiced
- 15 oz. can garbanzo beans, rinsed and drained
- 1/3 cup dried cranberries
- 1 avocado, pitted and diced
- 1/4 cup red onion, chopped
- 1/3 cup almonds, chopped
- 1/2 cup tahini
- 5 tablespoons warm water
- 1 teaspoon salt
- 1/4 teaspoon black pepper

Instructions:

1. Preheat the oven to 375F. Toss sweet potatoes with 2 teaspoons olive oil, 1/2 teaspoon salt, and 1/4 teaspoon pepper on a sheet pan. Bake for 40 minutes.
2. Add chopped kale, 1/2 lemon juice, 2 teaspoons olive oil, and 1/4 teaspoon salt to a bowl. Mix everything for 1 minute. Set aside.
3. Add tahini, 1 lemon juice, 1/4 teaspoon salt, and water to a bowl and whisk until creamy.
4. Add all ingredients together with kale and toss.Serve and enjoy.

SPRING VEGETABLE QUINOA MINESTRONE

Cook Time: 40 minutes

Servings: 6

Ingredients:

- 28 oz. can tomatoes, diced
- 1 tablespoon olive oil
- 3 garlic cloves, minced
- 1 cup carrots, sliced
- 1 white onion, diced
- 4 cups vegetable broth
- 2 teaspoons Italian seasoning
- 1/4 cup white quinoa, uncooked
- 2 bay leaves
- 1 cup zucchini, chopped
- 1 1/2 cups asparagus, chopped
- 1/2 cup frozen peas
- 1 cup packed kale, chopped
- 1 teaspoon nutritional yeast
- Salt and pepper, to taste

Instructions:

1. Add oil to a pan placed over medium-high heat. Add onions, carrots, and garlic and cook for 3 minutes. Add broth, quinoa, tomatoes, bay leaves, spices, salt, and pepper and mix well.
2. Bring to a boil, cover, reduce the heat and cook for 20 minutes.
3. Remove the lid and add the remaining vegetables. Cook for 10 minutes. Add seasoning to taste.Serve and enjoy.

CRANBERRY CILANTRO QUINOA SALAD

Cook Time: 15 minutes

Servings: 6

Ingredients:

- 1 1/2 cups vegetable broth
- 1 cup dry quinoa
- 1 lime juice
- 1/2 cup dried cranberries
- 4 tablespoons cilantro, chopped
- 1 1/2 teaspoon curry powder
- 1/2 cup bell pepper, diced
- 1/8 teaspoon cumin
- 1/4 cup green onions, chopped
- 1/3 cup almonds, toasted and sliced
- 1/2 cup carrots, grated
- 4 tablespoons pepitas
- 1 lime, cut into wedges
- olive oil
- Salt and pepper, to taste

Instructions:

1. Use a sieve to rinse and drain quinoa. Heat a saucepan over medium heat and toast quinoa.
2. Stir and toast for a few minutes. Add broth, turn the heat to high and bring to a boil.
3. Reduce the heat, cover and cook for 13 minutes. Mix cooked quinoa with cumin, lime juice, curry powder, pepitas, peppers, onions, almonds, and carrots. Season to taste and stir.
4. Chill and serve. Enjoy!

POWER LENTIL SOUP

Cook Time: 50 minutes

Servings: 4

Ingredients:

- 1 yellow onion, chopped
- 1/4 cup olive oil
- 4 garlic cloves, minced
- 2 carrots, peeled and chopped
- 2 teaspoons ground cumin
- 1/2 teaspoon dried thyme
- 1 teaspoon curry powder
- 28 oz. can tomatoes, diced
- 4 cups vegetable broth
- 1 cup green lentils, picked and rinsed
- 2 cups of water
- 1 cup kale
- 2 tablespoons lemon juice
- 1 teaspoon salt
- A pinch red pepper flakes
- black pepper, to taste

Instructions:

1. Heat olive oil in a pot over medium heat. Add carrot and chopped onion and cook for 5 minutes. Add cumin, garlic, curry powder and thyme. Cook for 30 seconds.

2. Add drained diced tomatoes and cook for a few minutes. Add water, broth, and lentils. Add 1 teaspoon salt and a pinch red pepper flakes — season with black pepper.

3. Increase the heat and bring the mixture to a boil, then cover and reduce the heat to simmer. Cook for 30 minutes. Transfer 2 cups to a blender and blend until smooth. Transfer back to pot.

4. Add chopped greens and cook for 5 minutes. Remove the pot from heat and add 1 tablespoon lemon juice.Serve and enjoy.

SWEET POTATO SALAD

Cook Time: 35 minutes

Servings: 4

Ingredients:

- 2 large sweet potatoes, peeled and cut into 1" cubes
- 1 tablespoon + 2 teaspoons olive oil
- 1/2 teaspoon paprika
- 1/2 teaspoon oregano
- 2 scallions, ends removed and diced
- 1 shallot, diced
- 3 tablespoons red wine vinegar
- 1 tablespoon maple syrup
- small bunch chives, chopped
- Salt and pepper, to taste

Instructions:

1. Preheat the oven to 390F and prepare a parchment-lined baking sheet.
2. Mix potato chunks with 1 tablespoon olive oil and spices. Place on the baking sheet and bake for 35 minutes. Let cool completely.
3. Add scallions, shallots, chives, maple syrup, vinegar and olive oil in a bowl. Add potatoes to the bowl.
4. Garnish with chives, refrigerate for 1 hour and serve.

ROASTED VEGETABLE SOUP WITH COUSCOUS

Cook time: 1 hour 20 minutes

Servings: 6

Ingredients:

- 2 medium carrots, peeled and chopped into 3/4" pieces
- 1 large onion, chopped
- 1 turnip, peeled and chopped into 3/4" pieces
- 1 sweet potato, chopped into 3/4" pieces
- 1 orange bell pepper, chopped into 3/4" pieces
- 1 head cauliflower, chopped into 1" florets
- 2 tablespoons olive oil
- 4 garlic cloves, minced
- 6 cups vegetable broth
- 15 oz. can diced tomatoes, fire-roasted
- 1/2 teaspoon dried rosemary
- 1/2 teaspoon dried thyme
- 15 oz. can cannellini beans, rinsed and drained
- 1/3 cup whole wheat couscous, uncooked
- parsley, chopped
- 1 teaspoon salt

- 1/2 teaspoon pepper

Instructions:

1. Preheat the oven to 425F and line a rimmed baking sheet with parchment paper.
2. Add onion, turnips, carrots, sweet potato, pepper, cauliflower and garlic to the baking pan. Add olive oil and toss. Spread in a layer. Bake for 15 minutes, stir and bake for another 15 minutes.
3. Transfer veggies to a pot. Add tomatoes, broth, rosemary, thyme, salt and pepper. Mix well. Turn the heat to medium high and bring to a simmer. Reduce the heat, cover and cook for 15 minutes.
4. Add beans and couscous and cook for 5 minutes. Serve topped with parsley.

FENNEL ASPARAGUS SALAD

Cook Time: 25 minutes

Servings: 4

Ingredients:

- 1/3 cup olive oil
- 1 large leek, white parts only
- 1 large fennel bulb
- 1 tablespoon lemon thyme
- 6 asparagus stalks
- 2 tablespoons lemon juice
- 1 teaspoon ground coriander
- 1 avocado, sliced
- 1/4 cup almonds, lightly toasted
- 3/4 teaspoon salt
- 1/2 teaspoon black pepper

Instructions:

1. Slice the white part of leek in circles. Add 3 tablespoon olive oil in a pan. Turn heat to medium and add leeks. Cook for 6 minutes. Season with salt and let cool.

2. Core and slice fennel bulbs into thin slices. Slice asparagus diagonally the same as fennel thickness and remove ends.
3. Add lemon juice, lemon thyme, coriander, remaining oil, salt and pepper in a bowl. Add fennel, leeks, and asparagus. Toss well.
4. Add almonds and avocado slices and serve.

SPICY ROASTED PARSNIP SOUP

Cook Time: 40 minutes

Servings: 4

Ingredients:

- 1 1/2 lbs parsnips, diced
- 2 tablespoons olive oil
- 1 teaspoon cumin seeds
- 1 teaspoon coriander seeds
- 1/2 teaspoon mustard seeds
- 1/2 teaspoon ground turmeric
- 1 onion, cut into 8 chunks
- 2 plum tomatoes, quartered
- 2 garlic cloves
- 1 tablespoon lemon juice
- 5 cups vegetable stock

Instructions:

1. Heat the oven to 425 F. Mix coriander seeds, turmeric, olive oil, cumin seeds, and mustard seeds in a bowl.

2. Add onions, parsnips, cloves, and tomatoes and mix well. Place on a heavy baking sheet and roast for 30 minutes.
3. Add to a blender with 2 1/2 cup vegetable stock and blend until smooth. Pour into the pan with remaining stock, season to taste and cook for 3-5 minutes.
4. Remove from heat and add lemon juice.Serve and enjoy.

FARRO TABBOULEH SALAD

Cook Time: 20 minutes

Servings: 4

Ingredients:

- 4 cups cooked faro
- 1/4 cup mint, chopped
- 1 bunch Italian parsley, chopped
- 1 English cucumber, diced
- 1 lb. cherry tomatoes, cut in half
- 1/4 cup olive oil
- 1/3 cup red onion, diced
- 1/8 cup lemon juice
- 3/4 teaspoon salt
- kalamata olives

Instructions:

1. Add mint cucumber, parsley, farro, tomatoes, and onions in a bowl and toss well to combine.
2. Add lemon juice and olive oil. Add salt to taste. Toss well to combine. Top with olives and serve. Enjoy!

MINTY PEA AND POTATO SOUP

Cook Time: 30 minutes

Servings: 4

Ingredients:

- 1 3/4 lbs potato, peeled and cut into chunks
- 2 teaspoons vegetable oil
- 4 1/5 cups vegetable stock
- 1 onion, chopped
- 4/5 lb frozen pea
- A handful mint, chopped

Instructions:

1. Heat oil in a pan and cook onions for 5 minutes.
2. Add stock and potatoes and bring to a boil. Cover and cook for 13 minutes, add peas and cook for 2 minutes more.
3. Remove ¼ of the veggies from the pan and set aside. Blend the remaining veggies and stock in a blender until smooth and mix with the reserved veggies, seasoning and mint.Serve and enjoy.

ITALIAN RICE NOODLES

Cook time: 20 minutes

Servings: 4

Ingredients

- 12 oz. rice noodles
- 3 pints small cherry tomatoes
- 2 large sprigs basil
- ¼ cup olive oil
- 1 red jalapeno, thinly sliced
- 6 garlic cloves, minced
- Kosher salt, to taste

Instructions

1. Add salted water to a saucepan and bring to a boil. Turn off the heat, then add the noodles. Let sit, stirring from time to time, for 4 minutes. Drain and rinse the noodles, then aside.

2. Add olive oil in a skillet and place over medium heat. Sauté garlic, frequently stirring, for 3 minutes. Stir in the basil sprigs and cook, stirring, for 1 minute. Add the cherry tomatoes and ¼ cup water and cook, infrequently stirring, for 10 minutes, then sprinkle with salt.

3. Toss noodles with sauce to coat, then serve. Enjoy!

MAPLE GLAZED TOFU

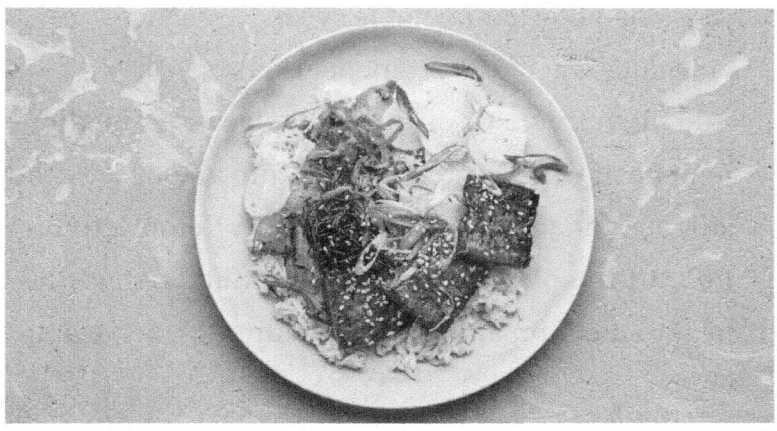

Cook time: 12 minutes

Servings: 2

Ingredients

- 1 block (12 oz.) firm tofu, drained
- 3 tablespoons maple syrup
- ¼ cup soy sauce
- 3 tablespoons rice vinegar
- ½ cup canola oil
- 1 ½-inch ginger, thinly sliced
- ½ teaspoon crushed red pepper flakes

Instructions

1. Drain the excess moisture from the tofu. Slice tofu into 9 pieces.

2. In a small bowl, mix maple syrup, soy sauce, rice vinegar, ginger, and red pepper flakes.

3. Add oil to a nonstick skillet and place over medium-high heat. Once heated up, add tofu and cook without stirring, for 4 minutes on each side. Remove tofu.

4. Pour the maple mixture into the skillet, reduce the heat to medium and cook for 4 minutes, serve and enjoy.

SPAGHETTI WITH KALE

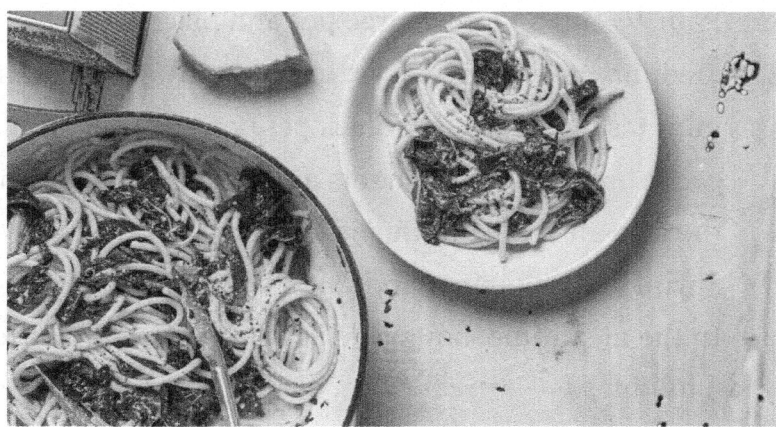

Cook time: 45 minutes

Servings: 4

Ingredients

- 12 oz spaghetti
- 3 bunches (1 ½ lb) kale, stem, and ribs removed, torn
- ¼ cup olive oil
- 5 garlic cloves, crushed
- Ground black pepper, to taste
- Salt, to taste

Instructions

1. Add salted water to a large pot and bring it to a boil. Add kale and cook for 2 minutes. Transfer kale to a

colander and rinse with cold water, then toss to remove excess liquid.

2. Pour ¼ cup oil into a large pot and place over medium heat. Sauté garlic, infrequently stirring, for 3 minutes. Sprinkle with black pepper and cook until garlic breaks into fragments and turn golden. Stir in the kale and cook, frequently stirring, for 8 minutes. Sprinkle with pepper and salt.

3. In the meantime, boil pasta in kale cooking water for 3 minutes.

4. Transfer pasta to the kale pot, then adds 1 cup pasta liquid. Cook, stirring and adding extra pasta liquid as needed, for 2 minutes. Season with black pepper and salt, serve.

LASAGNE (VEGAN VERSION)

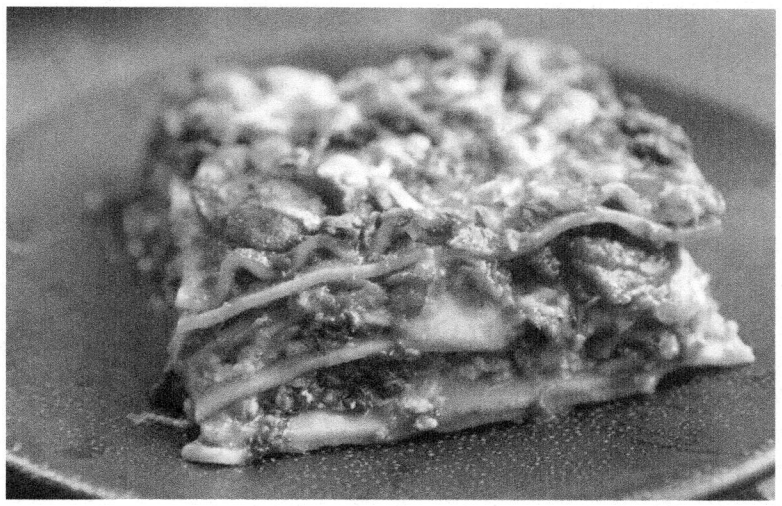

Cook time: 90 minutes

Servings: 6

Ingredients

- 10 dried egg-free lasagne sheets
- 9 oz. chestnut mushrooms, thinly sliced
- 3 ½ oz dried red lentils, split
- 2 (14 oz) tins tomatoes, chopped
- 5 ½ oz. spinach leaves
- 1 medium zucchini, sliced
- 1 small eggplant, sliced
- 4 tablespoons olive oil

- 1 cube vegetable stock, crumbled
- 1 onion, finely chopped
- 2 garlic cloves, crushed
- 1 red pepper, seeded, diced
- 2 teaspoons dried oregano
- 1 teaspoon sugar
- Ground black pepper and salt, to taste

  For the sauce:
- 1 ¼ pint almond milk
- 3 tablespoons sunflower oil
- 3 ½ oz. plain flour
- 3 tablespoons nutritional yeast flakes
- ¼ teaspoon ground nutmeg
- Ground black pepper and salt, to taste

Instructions

1. Preheat the oven to 400 F.
2. Sauté onion with olive oil, for 4 minutes, frequently stirring, in a large nonstick saucepan.
3. Stir in the mushrooms, eggplant, zucchini, and pepper, then sauté, frequently stirring, for 12 minutes. Add garlic and cook for some seconds.
4. Stir in the tomatoes, red lentils, vegetable stock, oregano, and sugar. Stir in 14 oz water into the pan, bring to a simmer and cook, frequently stirring, for 15

minutes. Add the spinach leaves to the pan and cook for 2 minutes.

5. Meanwhile, make the sauce by cooking the flour in hot oil, frequently stirring, for 1 minute, over medium heat. Add the milk, yeast, nutmeg, pepper and salt and cook, frequently stirring, for 5 minutes. Add more seasoning if necessary.

6. Prepare an ovenproof dish, layer 1/3 of the vegetable mixture on the bottom, then top with a layer of lasagne sheet. Add a second layer of the vegetable mixture on top and cover with another layer of lasagne sheet. Drizzle half of the sauce over and top with the remaining vegetable mixture — finally, layer with the remaining lasagne and sauce.

7. Bake for 40 minutes. Let stand for 5 minutes, cut and serve. Enjoy!

SPANISH VEGAN PAELLA

Cook time: 120 minutes

Servings: 6

Ingredients

For the sausage:

- 8 oz. vital wheat
- 2 tablespoons plain flour
- 1 oz. nutritional yeast flakes
- 3 ½ oz. dry sherry
- 1 cup vegetable stock
- 1 tablespoon tomato purée
- 2 tablespoons soy sauce
- 2 tablespoons olive oil
- ½ teaspoon ground fennel seeds
- 3 tablespoon smoked paprika
- 1 garlic clove, minced
- 1 teaspoon dried oregano
- 1 pinch cayenne pepper
- 1 teaspoon salt

For the paella:

- 5 oz tofu, crumbled
- 3 ½ ozgreen beans, chopped

- 1 lbpaella rice
- 8 small tomatoes, halved
- 2 ½ pints vegetable stock
- 26 oz. dry white wine
- 2 tablespoons olive oil
- 2 onions, finely chopped
- 3 peppers, chopped
- 4 garlic cloves, minced
- 1 teaspoon cayenne pepper
- 1 tablespoon paprika
- 1 pinch saffron
- Ground black pepper and salt, to taste

Instructions

For the sausage:

1. Combine all the wet ingredients in a bowl. Mix all the dry ingredients and stir them into the wet ingredients. Knead for 5 minutes to form firm dough.

2. Divide the dough into 2 parts and mold each half into a log shape. Place each log in the middle of a cling film. Roll the cling film around the log, then tighten into a sausage by twisting the ends of the cling film.

3. Pour water into a large saucepan, add the sausages and bring to a low simmer. Cook for an hour, adding more water if needed. Remove from the water and let

cool, then refrigerate overnight, without removing the wrapping.

For the paella:

1. Preheat the oven to 375 F. To a large saucepan, add the vegetable stock, white wine, and saffron. Stir and bring to a boil. Add the rice and simmer for 15 minutes on reduced heat, making sure to keep the rice wet by adding more vegetable broth if necessary.

2. In the meantime, sauté onion, pepper, and salt in a large paella pan placed over medium heat, for 5 minutes. Add in garlic and spices and sauté for 10 minutes. Add to the rice and stir to coat. Stir in the green beans and tomatoes. Add more vegetable stock if needed, then bake for 30 minutes.

3. Fry the sausage and tofu in oil, in a frying pan, over medium-high heat, for 4 minutes. Once the paella rice mixture is cooked, stir in the fried sausage and tofu. Serve in the pan.

ARTICHOKE MUSHROOM PIZZA

Cook time: 30 minutes

Servings: 4

Ingredients

- 7 oz. white bread flour, plus more for rolling
- 1½ teaspoon fast-action dried yeast
- ½ cup of warm water
- olive oil, for greasing
- 1 teaspoon caster sugar
- 1 teaspoon flaked sea salt

For the topping:

- 3 ½ oz. artichoke hearts in oil, drained, sliced
- 3 ½ oz. chestnut mushrooms, sliced
- 14 oz tin tomatoes, chopped
- ½ large zucchini, thinly sliced
- 16 black olives, drained
- 1 handful fresh basil leaves, torn
- 2 tablespoons olive oil
- 1 small onion, chopped
- ½ yellow pepper, seeded, sliced
- 2 garlic cloves, minced
- 4 tablespoons ground almonds
- 1 teaspoon dried oregano

- Ground black pepper and salt, to taste

Instructions

1. In a large bowl, mix the flour, yeast, sugar, and salt. Stir in water using a wooden spoon until a dough forms. Knead for 5 minutes on a work surface until smooth. Grease a bowl and place the dough inside, cover with an oiled cling film. Place in a warm place for about 1 hour.

2. Meanwhile, sauté onions in 2 tablespoons olive oil, over low heat, for 5 minutes, stirring constantly. Add the garlic after 4 minutes of cooking the onions. Stir in tomatoes, oregano, pepper, and salt. Increase heat to medium-high and cook, frequently stirring, for 10 minutes. Turn off the heat and leave to cool.

3. Divide the dough into two halves and mold into balls, flattening each ball slightly. Flour a rolling pin and a working surface, then roll out each ball until 10-inch in diameter.

4. Line non-stick baking papers on two separate baking trays, and place the dough on top. Top with the tomato mixture, leaving out the edges. Let stand for 40 minutes.

5. Preheat the oven to 425F. Top the pizzas with pepper, zucchini, mushrooms, artichoke, ground almonds,

and olives. Bake, one after another, for 10 minutes. Sprinkle with basil leaves and olive oil, then serve.

TOMATO CHILI BEAN

Cook time: 60 minutes

Servings: 8

Ingredients

- 14 oz tin black-eyed beans, drained, rinsed
- 14 oz can kidney beans, drained, rinsed
- 14 oz can borlotti beans, drained, rinsed
- 14 oz can butter beans, drained, rinsed
- 9 oz. mushrooms, chopped
- 2 tins (14 oz each) jackfruit in brine, drained, rinsed
- 1 lb tomato passata
- 14 oz tin plum tomatoes, squashed
- 3 celery sticks, chopped
- ½ tablespoon tomato purée
- 1 tablespoon coconut oil
- 1 teaspoon balsamic vinegar
- 2 onions, chopped
- 5 garlic cloves, minced
- 1 teaspoon tomato ketchup
- 2 teaspoons chili powder
- 1 teaspoon caster sugar
- Ground black pepper and salt, to taste

Instructions

1. In a large saucepan placed over medium heat, melt coconut oil and sauté onion and celery for 10 minutes. Stir in the mushrooms, garlic, and chili powder and cook for 10 minutes.
2. Add the jackfruit, chopped tomatoes, passata, and tomato puree. Stir and cook for a few more minutes.
3. In the meantime, combine vinegar, ketchup, and sugar in a small bowl, then add into the sauce. Stir in the beans and sprinkle with pepper and salt. Close the lid and cook for 40 minutes on low heat. Enjoy.

SWEET POTATO SQUASH WITH RICE

Cook time: 60 minutes

Servings: 4

Ingredients

- 1 lb. sweet potatoes, peeled, cut
- 1 large butternut squash, peeled, de-seeded, sliced
- 14 oz tin tomatoes, chopped
- 10 ½ oz. black rice, to serve
- 2 tablespoons vegetable oil
- 14 oz tin coconut milk
- 12 oz. vegetable stock
- 1 red onion, quartered
- 3 red chilies, stalks removed, cut into three
- 2 garlic cloves, halved
- 2 oz fresh ginger, peeled, thickly sliced
- 1 teaspoon ground turmeric
- ½ teaspoon ground cinnamon
- 1 teaspoon ground coriander
- 1 teaspoon of sea salt

Instructions

1. In a food processor, pulse onions, chilies, garlic, ginger, ground coriander, turmeric, cinnamon, and salt until processed.

2. Heat olive oil in a casserole dish. Add the onion mixture and sauté, stirring properly, for 1 minute.

3. Stir in the vegetable stock, coconut milk, tinned tomatoes, squash, and potato, then bring to a boil. Reduce the heat, close the lid and simmer for 50 minutes. Add more seasoning if needed. Remove from heat and let stand for 10 minutes.

4. In the meantime, cook rice according to package instructions. Then serve with potato mixture.

CURRY BEANS

Cook time: 30 minutes

Servings: 4

Ingredients

- 4 ½ oz. French beans
- 4 ½ oz. zucchini, cut into chunks
- 4 ½ oz. sweet potatoes, peeled, cubed
- 4 ½ oz. pumpkin, peeled, cubed
- 14 oz tin coconut milk
- 3 ½ oz. vegetable stock
- 1 bunch spring onions, sliced

For the curry paste:

- 10 black peppercorns
- 6 lemongrass stalks
- 1 lime, zested
- 2 ½ tablespoon vegetable oil
- 1 splash chili oil
- 2 teaspoons coriander seeds
- 2 teaspoons cumin seeds
- 5 shallots
- 4 red chilies
- ½-inch piece fresh ginger, peeled

- 2 garlic cloves, crushed
- ½ teaspoon turmeric
- 1 pinch ground cinnamon
- 1 tablespoon sugar
- Salt, to taste
- Basmati rice, cooked

Instructions

1. For the curry paste: place a skillet over medium heat and fry the peppercorns, coriander and cumin seeds, without oil, until fragrant, then grind them in a mortar.
2. Place them and the other paste ingredients (apart from oil) into a food processor and process for 5 minutes.
3. Heat the oil in a frying pan and sauté 4 teaspoons curry paste until fragrant. Stir in the vegetable stock and coconut milk and simmer for 3 minutes in high heat. Add pumpkin, potatoes, and onions and cook for extra 5 minutes. Add beans and zucchini, then simmer for 5 minutes.
4. Enjoy with the cooked rice.

FRIED TOFU AND EDAMAME

Cook time: 10 minutes

Servings: 4

Ingredients

For the fried tofu:

- 14 oz. firm tofu, drained and sliced
- 3 tablespoons light soy sauce
- 1 teaspoon dark soy sauce
- 2 tablespoons groundnut oil
- 1 tablespoon balsamic vinegar
- 1 teaspoon dried chili flakes

For the edamame beans:

- 3 oz. frozenedamamebeans, defrosted
- 1 handful fresh coriander, chopped
- 1 tablespoon groundnut oil
- 1 teaspoon light soy sauce
- 1 teaspoon balsamic vinegar
- 1 red chili, de-seeded, finely chopped

Instructions

1. For the fried tofu, sauté tofu in groundnut oil, in a frying pan, for 3 minutes. Stir in the light soy and

cook until the liquid has reduced. Flip the tofu over and cook for an extra 3 minutes.

2. Pour in the dark soy sauce and balsamic vinegar, then cook until the liquid is reduced to half. Sprinkle with chili flakes, to taste. Transfer the tofu to a serving plate and set aside.

3. To cook the edamame, sauté red chili in groundnut oil for a few seconds. Add the edamame beans and 1 tsp. water, then cook for 1 minute. Drizzle with the balsamic vinegar and light soy sauce, then add the chopped coriander and stir.

4. Top the tofu with the beans and enjoy.

CHILI SPAGHETTI

Cook time: 30 minutes

Servings: 4

Ingredients

- 14 oz. spaghetti, cooked, drained
- 1 tablespoon flat-leaf parsley, chopped
- 5 tablespoons olive oil
- 3 garlic cloves, minced
- 3 fresh red chilies, seeded, chopped
- Salt, to taste

Instructions

1. Sauté chilies and garlic in olive oil, for 3-4 minutes.
2. Add the cooked spaghetti and toss to coat.
3. Top with parsley, sprinkle with salt, and serve. Enjoy!

FRENCH STEWED VEGETABLE (RATATOUILLE)

Cook time: 60 minutes

Servings: 4

Ingredients

- 4 large tomatoes, peeled, seeded, chopped
- 4 small zucchini, sliced
- 2 eggplants, quartered lengthwise, sliced
- Small bunch basil, torn
- 4 tablespoons olive oil
- 2 onions, chopped
- 2 red peppers, seeded, chopped
- 2 garlic cloves, crushed
- ½ teaspoon sugar
- Ground black pepper and salt, to taste

Instructions

1. Sauté onions in oil, stirring often, for 10 minutes. Stir in the zucchini and eggplants, increase the heat a bit and sauté for 3 minutes.
2. Add garlic, red pepper, sugar, ground pepper, salt and half of the basil. Stir, reduce the heat to a gentle simmer, cover and cook for 20 minutes.
3. Mix in the tomatoes and cook for 10 minutes. Sprinkle with the remaining basil and serve. Enjoy!

SPINACH PUREE AND SAUTÉED CHICKPEA

Cook time: 30 minutes

Servings: 4

Ingredients

- 7 oz. canned chickpeas, drained, rinsed
- 2 lbs fresh spinach
- 14 oz. tinned tomatoes, chopped
- 1 eggplant, sliced
- 2 tablespoons olive oil
- 2 medium red onions, chopped
- 2 hot green chilies, halved, sliced, not seeded
- 2 garlic cloves, minced
- 1 tablespoon cumin seeds
- 1 tablespoon coriander seeds, ground
- Salt, to taste

Instructions

1. Bring water to a boil, then cook spinach in it for 2 minutes. Rinse with cold water and drain. Place in a food processor and process until almost smooth. Set aside.

2. Sauté onions, chickpeas, garlic, chili and spices in half olive oil, over medium heat, for 5 minutes.

3. Pour in the remaining olive oil, then add the eggplant and cook, constantly stirring, for 10 minutes. Stir in the tomatoes, add a pinch of salt. Reduce the heat, cover and cook for 15 minutes. Mix in the spinach puree and serve.

PASTA WITH BEANS

Cook time: 20 minutes

Servings: 4

Ingredients

- 12 oz. spaghetti, cooked, reserve ½ cup cooking the liquid
- 1 can (15 oz.) cannellini beans, drained, rinsed
- 1 cup green pesto

Instructions

1. In a bowl, toss spaghetti with pesto, reserved cooking liquid, and beans. Enjoy!

VEGAN ENCHILADAS

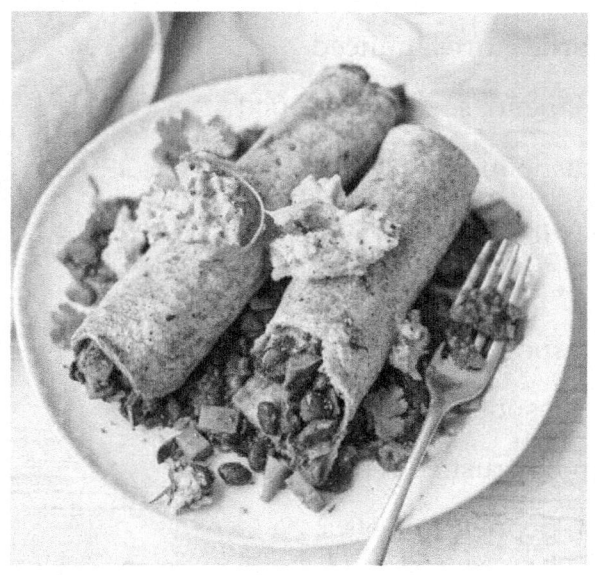

Cook time: 70 minutes

Servings: 8

Ingredients

- 8 (8-inch) flour tortillas
- 1 (15 oz.) can black beans, rinsed
- 1 (28 oz.) can tomatoes, diced
- 1 large Russet potato, sliced
- 1 large sweet potato, sliced
- 1 cup cheese, shredded

- 6 tablespoons olive oil
- 1 yellow onion, chopped
- 2 garlic cloves, minced
- 1 jalapeño, seeded, chopped
- 1 teaspoon cumin
- 1 teaspoon smoked paprika
- 1/2 teaspoon dried Mexican oregano
- 1 teaspoon sugar
- 1 tablespoon chili powder
- 1 pinch crushed red pepper
- Salt, pepper, to taste

Instructions

1. Preheat the oven to 350°F. In a bowl, combine potatoes, ¼ cup olive oil, sprinkle with black pepper and salt, and toss well. Transfer to a baking sheet and roast for 50 minutes.

2. Sauté onion in 2 tablespoons oil over medium heat for 7 minutes. Stir in the garlic, jalapeno, cumin, paprika, oregano, crushed red pepper, sugar, chili powder, black pepper, and salt. Cook, stirring, for 1 minute. Tip the tomatoes.

3. Turn off the heat and blend using an immersion blender until pureed. Turn on the heat and cook for 20 minutes.

4. In a bowl, toss the potatoes with the beans and 1 cup sauce.

5. Microwave the tortillas, wrapped in damp paper towels, for 1 minute. Top with ½ cup potato mixture and roll-up.

6. Layer some sauce on the bottom of a glass baking dish. Line with the tortillas. Sprinkle with the remaining sauce and cheese. Bake for 20 minutes and serve.

STUFFED PEPPERS

Cook time: 40 minutes

Servings: 4

Ingredients

- ¾ lb oyster mushrooms, sliced
- 4 cups spinach, chopped
- 1/4 cup Thai basil, chopped
- 3/4 cup long-grain white rice
- 1/2 cup unsweetened coconut milk
- 2 tablespoons unsalted butter
- 1 tablespoon fresh lemon juice
- 2 medium shallots, minced
- 4 garlic cloves, minced
- 4 large bell peppers
- 1 jalapeño, chopped
- 1 tablespoon ginger, minced
- 1 tablespoon Thai red curry paste
- Salt, to taste

Instructions

1. Boil a pot of water. Cut off the pepper tops, remove the stems and cores, dice the tops. Cook the hollowed out peppers in hot water for 4 minutes. Transfer to paper towels and place cut side down to drain. Save 1 ½ cups of the cooking water and discard the rest.

2. Melt 1 tablespoon butter in a saucepan over medium heat. Add the garlic, shallots, and salt and cook for 3 minutes. Add the rice and cook for 4 minutes, stirring. Mix in the coconut milk, curry paste, 1 ½ cups pepper water, and ginger, then bring to a simmer. Reduce the heat to low and cook, covered, for 25 minutes.

3. In the meantime, preheat the oven to 350°F. Melt 1 tablespoon butter in a skillet, over medium heat. Sauté the jalapeno and the diced pepper tops for 5 minutes, stirring frequently. Stir in the mushrooms, cover and cook, stirring, for 5 minutes. Cook for extra 4 minutes, uncovered, stirring. Add spinach and cook for 1 minute.

4. Toss the vegetable mixture with the rice mixture. Add lemon juice, basil and salt then stir to combine. Stuff the peppers with the rice mixture and place them on a glass baking dish. Bake, covered with foil, for 45 minutes. Serve and enjoy.

FRIED PAD THAI RICE NOODLES

Cook time: 15 minutes

Servings: 4

Ingredients

- 1/2 lb dried pad Thai rice noodles
- 2 cups (3/4 lb) julienned carrots
- 1/4 cup soy sauce
- 1 tablespoon tamarind paste
- 2 tablespoons vegetable oil
- 1 tablespoon Sriracha
- 4 scallions, sliced
- 2 garlic cloves, minced
- 2 small shallots, sliced
- 2 tablespoons light brown sugar

Instructions

1. Soak the noodles in very hot water for 15 minutes. Drain and remove any excess liquid.
2. In the meantime,combine soy sauce, tamarind paste, Sriracha, and brown sugar in a bowl.

3. Heat oil in a large nonstick skillet over high heat, then sauté carrots, shallots, and garlic, infrequently stirring, for 5 minutes. Add the noodles and scallions and cook, stirring, for 2 minutes.
4. Pour in the soy sauce mixture and cook, stirring, for 3 minutes. Transfer to a serving platter and enjoy.

JUICY SAUTÉED MUSHROOMS AND CORN

Cook time: 15 minute

Servings: 6

Ingredients

- 6 medium dried shiitake mushroom caps
- 10 ears white corn, shucked
- 2 tablespoons olive oil
- 1 tablespoon fresh lemon juice
- 2 medium shallots, minced
- 1 teaspoon lemon zest, finely grated
- 1 garlic clove, minced
- Ground black pepper and salt, to taste

Instructions

1. Soak the mushrooms in boiling water for 15 minutes.
2. In the meantime, grate 5 ears of corn down to the cob on the coarse side of the grater. Cut the kernels from the other ears of corn using a serrated knife. Scrape the cobs juices into the bowl using the dull side of the knife.

3. Drain and cut the mushrooms into pieces. Sauté the mushrooms, garlic, and shallots in heated oil, stirring from time to time, for 10 minutes. Increase the heat to high. When the oil starts sizzling, stir in the corn and corn juice and cook, stirring, for 3 minutes. Drizzle with the lemon juice, sprinkle with lemon zest, pepper and salt, then serve.

SAFFRON QUINOA WITH PISTACHIOS

Cook time: 15 minutes

Servings: 4

Ingredients

- 1 1/2 cups quinoa
- 1/3 cup dried apricots, chopped
- 1/3 cup roasted salted shelled pistachios, chopped
- 4 green cardamom pods, cracked
- 2 tablespoons olive oil
- 1 medium onion, chopped
- 1/4 teaspoon ground turmeric
- 4 saffron threads
- Fine Himalayan pink salt

Instructions

1. Sauté onions and salt in olive oil over medium heat, stirring from time to time, for 7 minutes. Stir in the quinoa, apricots, cardamom, saffron and turmeric and stir-fry for 2 minutes. Pour in 3 cups of water and bring to a boil. Simmer over low heat, covered, for 20 minutes.

2. Turn off the heat and leave, covered, for 20 minutes. Discard the cardamom pods, then fluff the quinoa using a fork. Stir in the pistachios and sprinkle with salt, then serve.

SAUTÉED CABBAGE

Cook time: 20 minutes

Servings: 6

Ingredients

- 3 lbsgreen cabbage, cored, shredded
- 2 tablespoons olive oil
- 1 ½ teaspoon cumin seeds
- 1 ½ teaspoons turmeric
- 1 ½ teaspoon kosher salt

Instructions

1. Sauté cumin seeds in olive oil, over medium heat, for 30 seconds.
2. Mix in the cabbage, turmeric and salt and cook for 20 minutes, stirring from time to time. Enjoy.

FRIED RICE

Cook time: 60 minutes

Servings: 4

Ingredients

For rice and vegetables:

- 1 cup (8 oz.) extra-firm tofu
- 1 cup brown rice, rinsed, boiled
- 1/2 cup carrots, finely diced
- 1/2 cup peas
- 4 garliccloves, minced
- 1 cup green onion, chopped

For sauce:

- 4 tablespoons tamari
- 2 teaspoons chili garlic sauce
- 1 tablespoon peanut butter
- 3 tablespoons brown sugar
- 1 garlicclove, minced

Instructions

1. Preheat the oven to 400°F. Grease a baking sheet with non-stick cooking spray.

2. Meanwhile, wrap tofu in a towel then drain the liquid by placing something heavy on top. Dice the tofu and transfer it to the baking sheet. Bake for 30 minutes and set aside.

3. In the meantime, whisk all the sauce ingredients in a bowl (except 1 tablespoons tamari). When the tofu is cooked, soak in the sauce, infrequently stirring, for 5 minutes.

4. Place a large skillet over medium heat. When it gets hot, transfer the tofu to the skillet, leaving the sauce behind. Cook, infrequently stirring, for 4 minutes, then transfer to a plate.

5. Sauté carrots, peas, onions, and garlic, infrequently stirring, for 4 minutes. Drizzle with 1 tablespoon tamari. Stir in the rice, tofu and the remaining tamari. Cook, constantly stirring, for 4 minutes, over medium-high heat. Serve and enjoy.

ZUCCHINI BALLS WITH PASTA

Cook time: 25 minutes

Servings: 4

Ingredients

- 1 (15 oz.) can chickpeas, drained, rinsed
- 1 zucchini, shredded
- 1/2 cup rolled oats
- 8 oz. whole grain pasta
- 32 oz. marinara sauce
- 1/2 lemon, juiced
- 3 garlic cloves
- 1 teaspoon dried basil
- 1 teaspoon dried oregano
- 2 tablespoons nutritional yeast
- 1/2 teaspoon salt

Instructions

1. Pulse chickpeas rolled oats and garlic cloves in a food processor for 10 seconds. Transfer to a large bowl, then mix with 1 cup zucchini, nutritional yeast, dried herbs, and lemon juice.

2. Preheat the oven to 375°F. Divide and roll the zucchini mixture into 12 separate balls, then place them on a baking sheet lined with parchment paper.

3. Bake for 25 minutes. In the meantime, cook pasta according to package instructions. Serve the zucchini balls with the pasta and marinara sauce.

SLOPPY JOES

Cook time: 25 minutes

Servings: 4

Ingredients

For lentils:

- 1 cup green lentils, rinsed
- 2 cups of water
  For sloppy joes:
- 1 (15 oz.) can tomato sauce
- 2 tablespoons vegan Worcestershire sauce
- 2 tablespoons olive oil
- 1/2 medium white onion, minced
- 1/2 medium green bell pepper, diced
- 2 garlic cloves, minced
- 2 teaspoons chili powder
- 1 teaspoon ground cumin
- 2 tablespoons coconut sugar
- Ground black pepper and salt, to taste

Instructions

1. Add 2 cups water and lentils to a saucepan and bring to a boil over medium-high heat. Lower the heat to a simmer and cook for 18 minutes, uncovered. Drain and set aside.
2. Sauté onions, bell pepper, garlic, a pinch of black pepper and salt in olive oil, constantly stirring, for 5 minutes.
3. Mix in the tomato sauce, Worcestershire sauce, coconut sugar, cumin, and chili powder. Stir in the cooked lentils and cook over medium-low heat for 10 minutes. Serve.

MUSHROOM RISOTTO

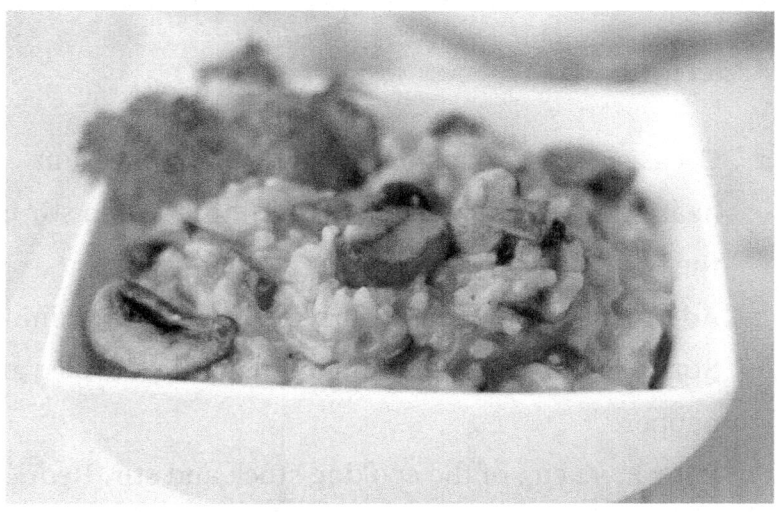

Cook time: 30 minutes

Servings: 4

Ingredients

- 1 cup white Arborio rice, uncooked
- 1 tablespoon fresh mint, chopped
- 3 cups vegetable stock
- 1 cup beet puree
- 1/2 cup sweet onion, chopped
- 1 teaspoon garlic, minced
- 1/2 teaspoon cinnamon

- 1/4 teaspoon allspice
- 1/4 teaspoon black pepper

Instructions

1. Grease a cast-iron skillet and place over medium heat. Add onion and cook for 3 minutes, then stir in the beets.
2. Add the rice and let it absorb the liquid for 3 minutes. Stir in the mint leaves, cinnamon, garlic, allspice and pepper.
3. Pour in ½ cup of the cooking stock and stir. Reduce the heat to medium-low and let the rice absorb the liquid. Repeat the process (without reducing the heat further) until the vegetable stock is all absorbed. Serve and enjoy.

MILKY CAULIFLOWER PASTA

Cook time: 30 minutes

Servings: 5

Ingredients

- 3 ½ cups (12 oz.) cauliflower florets
- 3/4 cup raw cashews, chopped
- 1lb whole wheat pasta
- 3 ½ cups plain almond milk
- 3 tablespoons yellow miso
- ½ tablespoon white vinegar
- ½ tablespoon tomato paste
- ¼ cup of coconut oil
- 2 garlic cloves, sliced
- 2 tablespoons nutritional yeast
- 2 teaspoons ground mustard
- 1 teaspoon salt

Instructions

1. Cook tomato paste, nutritional yeast, mustard, garlic and salt in hot olive oil over medium heat, stirring, for 45 seconds. Stir in the almond milk and bring to a simmer, scraping the pot bottom with a wooden

spoon.

2. Add the cauliflower, cashew, and miso, reduce the heat to medium-low and cook, partially covered and infrequently stirring, for 20 minutes.

3. Using an immersion blender, blend the mixture until properly blended, then set aside.

4. In the meantime, cook pasta according to package instructions in well-salted water. Drain the pasta, reserving ½ cup of the cooking liquid.

5. Add the cooked pasta into the cauliflower sauce and stir. Stir in vinegar and a splash of the pasta liquid. Cook on medium-low heat until the sauce has thickened out. Sprinkle with pepper and salt to taste, then serve.

POTATO CHIPS

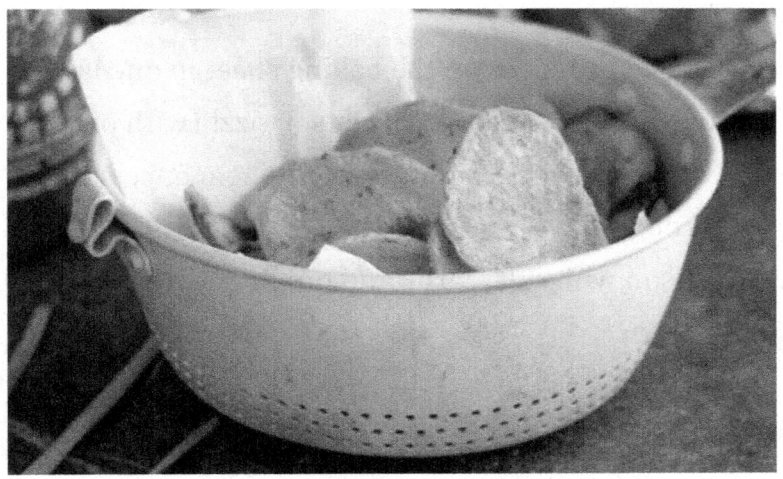

Cooking time: 20 minutes

Servings: 4-6

Ingredients:

- 3 potatoes, cleaned
- 2 tablespoons extra-virgin olive oil
- 1 teaspoon sea salt, or to taste
- ¼ teaspoon onion powder
- ¼ teaspoon garlic powder
- A pinch of chili powder

Instructions:

1. Preheat the oven to 400 F.

2. Thinly slice the potatoes. Soak in warm water for about 10-15 minutes. Drain well and pat the slices dry.

3. Spread the slices on the baking sheet in one layer, and you may need two sheets. Drizzle with oil and bake for about 20 minutes. Flip them once halfway through.

4. Season with salt, garlic and onion powders and chili powder.

CRACKERS WITH EDAMAME HUMMUS

Cooking time: 5 minutes

Servings: 6-8

Ingredients:

- 1 cup edamame, frozen, thawed, shelled
- 3 ½ tablespoons tahini
- 2 garlic cloves, chopped
- 2 tablespoons lemon juice
- 2 tablespoons olive oil
- 3 tablespoons water
- ¼ teaspoon onion powder
- Whole-wheat crackers
- Vegetable slices (bell peppers, celery, cucumber)
- Salt, pepper, to taste

Instructions:

1. Add edamame, tahini, garlic, lemon juice, oil, water, onion powder, salt, and pepper to a blender and blitz well until smooth.
2. Cover and refrigerate for 1 hour.
3. Serve with crackers and veggies.

PEANUT BUTTER JELLY APPLE NACHOS

Cooking time: 5 minutes

Servings: 2

Ingredients:

- 2 apples
- 4 tablespoons jelly of choice
- 4 tablespoons peanut butter
- Chia seeds, for serving

Instructions:

1. Slice the apples and place them on a large plate.
2. Top with jelly and peanut butter. Sprinkle with chia seeds and serve. Enjoy!

FRIED CINNAMON BANANAS

Cooking time: 5 minutes

Servings: 2

Ingredients:

- 2 bananas, peeled and sliced
- 1 teaspoon cinnamon
- 2 tablespoons sugar
- ¼ teaspoon nutmeg

Instructions:

1. Mix cinnamon, sugar and nutmeg in a bowl.
2. Preheat a skillet over medium heat, coat with cooking spray. Add banana and top with the sugar mixture.
3. Cook for 2-3 minutes per side. Serve and enjoy!

MAPLE ALMOND POPCORN

Cooking time: 5 minutes

Servings: 4

Ingredients:

- 1/2 cup corn kernels
- 1 cup roasted almonds
- 1/4 cup coconut oil
- 2 tablespoons maple syrup
- 2 tablespoons cane sugar
- 1/2 teaspoon sea salt

Instructions:

1. Preheat oil in a pan over medium heat. Add the corn and stir well to coat in oil.
2. Add maple syrup and sugar, cover with the lid.
3. When the corn starts popping, shake the pan. Keep shaking from time to time. Cook until you heat almost no popping sounds.
4. Add sea salt and serve.

TURMERIC SNACK BALLS

Cooking time: 10 minutes

Servings: 8-10

Ingredients:

- 1/2 cup walnuts
- 8 Medjool dates, pitted, chopped
- 1/2 cup shredded coconut, unsweetened
- 1 tablespoon unsweetened cocoa powder
- 1 teaspoon ground turmeric
- 1/2 teaspoon ground cinnamon

Instructions:

1. Add walnuts, dates, coconut, cocoa powder, turmeric, and cinnamon to a blender or a food processor and blitz until combined and the mixture sticks together.
2. Shape the mixture to balls and place them into a container. Refrigerate before serving. Enjoy!

HERBED FINGERLING POTATOES

Cooking time: 30 minutes

Servings: 4-6

Ingredients:

- 1 ½ lb fingerling potatoes, cleaned
- 1 cup vegetable broth
- 1 tablespoon fresh chives
- 1 tablespoon marjoram
- 1 teaspoon garlic powder
- 1 tablespoon thyme
- 1 teaspoon onion flakes
- 1 teaspoon rosemary
- Sea salt, pepper, to taste

Instructions:

1. Add potatoes to a pan and cover with water. Bring to a boil and cook for about 20 minutes, partially covered, until tender.
2. Add broth to a separate pan along with marjoram, thyme, rosemary, onion flakes, and garlic powder.

Cover and let rest while the potatoes are being cooked.

3. Drain the potatoes and rinse with cold. Half them lengthwise.
4. Bring the broth to a boil and add the potatoes. Cook for about 5 minutes, stirring from time to time.
5. Season with salt and pepper, and sprinkle with chives. Serve and enjoy!

GRILLED PORTOBELLO MUSHROOMS

Cooking time: 8 minutes

Servings: 4

Ingredients:

- 4 portobello mushrooms, stemmed
- 3 garlic cloves, minced
- 3 tablespoons low-sodium soy sauce
- 3 tablespoons brown rice syrup
- 1 tablespoon ginger, grated
- Salt, pepper, to taste

Instructions:

1. Mix the garlic, ginger, soy sauce, brown rice syrup, salt, and pepper in a bowl.
2. Place the mushrooms into the baking dish and pour the mixture over them — coat well and marinate for 1 hour.
3. Preheat the grill to medium-high heat. Place the mushrooms on the grill and cook for 4 minutes per side.
4. Serve and enjoy!

JORDANIAN SPICED ROASTED CHICKPEAS

Cooking time: 40 minutes

Servings: 4

Ingredients:

- 1 ½ cups chickpeas, cooked
- ½ tablespoon garlic powder
- ½ tablespoon onion powder
- A pinch of ground black pepper
- A pinch of ground turmeric
- A pinch of paprika

Instructions:

1. Preheat the oven to 400°F. Prepare a baking sheet and line it with parchment paper.
2. Mix garlic powder, onion powder, turmeric, black pepper and paprika in a bowl.
3. Spread the chickpeas on the baking sheet in one layer. Season with the spice mixture and toss well to coat.
4. Bake for 25 minutes. Stir the chickpeas and bake for 15 minutes more. Serve and enjoy!

SPICY FRENCH FRIES

Cooking time: 35 minutes

Servings: 4-6

Ingredients:

- 4 russet potatoes, cut into wedges 1 inch thick
- 1 lemon, juiced
- 1 tablespoon onion powder
- 1 teaspoon ground turmeric
- 1 teaspoon ground coriander
- 1 ½ teaspoon garlic powder
- 1 ½ teaspoon sweet paprika
- ¼ teaspoon cayenne pepper
- Sea salt, to taste

Instructions:

1. Preheat the oven to 450°F. Prepare a baking sheet and line it with parchment paper.
2. Add about 2 inches water to a pot and place the steamer basket on top. Place over medium heat and add the potato wedges to the basket.
3. Cover and steam for about 10 minutes. Transfer to a bowl.

4. Mix all the spices in a bowl. Add the spice mixture to potatoes and toss well to coat. Spread the wedges on the baking sheet in one layer and bake for 20-25 minutes.
5. Serve and enjoy!

CRUSTED ASPARAGUS SPEARS

Cooking time: 25 minutes

Servings: 4

Ingredients:

- 1 bunch asparagus, washed and trimmed
- 1/4 cup whole-wheat breadcrumbs
- 3 garlic cloves, minced
- 2 tablespoons hemp seeds
- ½ lemon, juiced
- 1/4 cup nutritional yeast
- 1/8 teaspoon ground pepper
- A pinch of paprika

Instructions:

1. Preheat the oven to 350°F. Prepare a baking sheet and line it with parchment paper.
2. Mix the hemp seeds, garlic, breadcrumbs, nutritional yeast, pepper and paprika in a bowl.
3. Place the asparagus on the baking sheet in one layer. Sprinkle with the hemp seeds mixture.
4. Bake for 20-25 minutes until asparagus are crispy. Sprinkle with lemon juice and serve. Enjoy!

BUFFALO CAULIFLOWER BITES

Cooking time: 25 minutes

Servings: 6

Ingredients:

- 1 head cauliflower, chopped into florets
- ⅔ cup brown rice flour
- 2 tablespoons almond flour
- ⅓ cup vegan hot sauce
- 2/3 cup water
- 1 tablespoon tomato paste
- 2 teaspoons onion powder
- 2 teaspoons garlic powder
- 1 teaspoon dried parsley
- 2 teaspoons smoked paprika

Instructions:

1. Preheat the oven to 450°F. Prepare two baking sheets and line them with parchment paper.
2. Mix rice flour, almond flour, garlic powder, onion powder, paprika, parsley, water, and tomato paste in a blender. Blitz until the mixture is smooth and thick.

3. Put the cauliflower florets into a bowl, add the mixture from the blender and toss well to coat.

4. Spread the florets on the baking sheets in one layer — Bake for 20-25 minutes.

5. Let rest for about 5 minutes and transfer to a bowl. Drizzle with hot sauce. Serve and enjoy!

VEGAN 'BACON' STRIPS

Cooking time: 50 minutes

Servings: 16

Ingredients:

- ½ eggplant, cut into strips
- 1 tablespoon vegan Worcestershire sauce
- ½ tablespoon maple syrup
- 1 tablespoon soy sauce
- 1 teaspoon smoked paprika
- 1 ½ tablespoons olive oil
- A pinch of ground cumin

Instructions:

1. Preheat the oven to 250°F. Prepare two baking sheets and line them with parchment paper.
2. Mix soy sauce, oil, Worcestershire sauce, maple syrup and cumin in a bowl.
3. Spread the eggplant sticks on the baking sheets in one layer and brush with the mixture from both sides.
4. Roast for about 45-50 minutes. Let cool slightly before serving. Serve and enjoy!

FUDGY DOUBLE CHOCOLATE APPLE MUFFINS

Cooking time: 22 minutes

Servings: 12

Ingredients:

- 1 1/3 cups whole-wheat flour
- 1 cup applesauce, unsweetened
- 2 flax eggs
- 1/3 cup dairy-free chocolate chips
- 1/4 cup maple syrup
- 1/4 cup coconut oil, melted
- 1/4 cup unsweetened almond milk
- 1/3 cup brown sugar
- 1/4 teaspoon sea salt
- 1 ½ teaspoons baking soda
- 1/2 cup unsweetened cocoa powder

Instructions:

1. Preheat the oven to 375°F. Prepare a muffin tin and line the cups with paper liners.

2. Mix applesauce, coconut oil, maple syrup, brown sugar, baking soda and salt in a bowl and stir well to combine.
3. Add the milk and mix well. Add the flours and cocoa powder, stir well until smooth.
4. Add the chocolate chips and pour the batter into the muffin cups and bake for 20-22 minutes.
5. Let cool before serving and enjoy!

SALTED CARAMEL APPLE BARS

Cooking time: 30 minutes

Servings: 10

Ingredients:

- 2 apples, grated
- 3/4 cup Medjool dates, pitted
- 2/3 cup tahini
- 1 cup oat flour
- 1 cup rolled oats
- 1/4 cup + 2 tablespoons unsweetened almond milk
- 3 tablespoons chia seeds
- 1 teaspoon vanilla extract
- 1 teaspoon baking powder
- 1/2 teaspoon salt

Instructions:

1. Preheat the oven to 350 F.
2. Mix oat flour, rolled oats, baking powder and salt in a bowl. Stir until well combined.
3. Add the dates, tahini, chia seeds, almond milk and vanilla extract to a blender or a food processor. Blitz until smooth.

4. Add the mixture to the flour mixture along with apples, stir well until combined.
5. Spread the batter into a baking pan, bake for about 30 minutes.
6. Let cool and cut into bars. Serve and enjoy!

LEMON CHEESECAKE

Cooking time: 15 minutes + chilling time

Servings: 6

Ingredients:

- 7 oz digestive biscuits, crushed
- 3 oz vegan margarine, melted
- 1 block (14 oz) firm tofu
- 1 tablespoon vegan cream cheese
- 1 can (14 oz) coconut cream
- ¼ lb caster sugar
- 1 lemon, zested and juiced
- ¾ cup limoncello
- 2-3 drops vanilla extract
- 3 tablespoons agar-agar
- Berries or fruits of choice, for serving

Instructions:

1. Combine the biscuits and margarine in a bowl. Transfer the mixture to a springform pan and press it into the bottom.
2. Mix lemon juice, agar-agar and limoncello in a pan and place over low heat. Add a splash of water if the

mixture is too thick. Stir until the mixture is smooth and agar is dissolved.

3. Add tofu, cream cheese, sugar, lemon zest, coconut cream, and vanilla to a blender and blitz well until smooth.

4. Pour the mixture over the crust and spread evenly. Refrigerate for 1 hour and serve topped with fruits or/and berries. Enjoy!

LEMON-OATMEAL COOKIES

Cooking time: 45 minutes

Servings: 7-8

Ingredients:

- 1/2 cup rolled oats
- 1/2 cup oat flour
- 1/4 cup quick-cooking oats
- 4-5 dates, pitted
- 1/2 cup applesauce, unsweetened
- 3/4 teaspoon apple cider vinegar
- 1/3 cup walnuts, chopped
- 1 lemon, zested
- 1 teaspoon of cocoa powder
- 1/2 teaspoon vanilla powder
- 1/4 teaspoon baking soda
- A pinch of salt

Instructions:

1. Preheat the oven to 275 F. Prepare a baking sheet and line it with parchment paper.
2. Soak dates in hot water for about 20 minutes. Drain and add to a blender.

3. Add vinegar and applesauce and blitz until a paste is formed.

4. Combine rolled oats, oat flour, quick-cooking oats, walnuts, lemon zest, cocoa powder, vanilla powder, baking soda and salt in a bowl. Add the date mixture and mix well.

5. Shape the mixture into balls and place them on the baking sheet. Press slightly.

6. Bake for 35-45 minutes. Let cool before serving. Enjoy!

COCONUT CHOCOLATE MOUSSE

Cooking time: 10 minutes

Servings: 2

Ingredients:

- Coconut cream from 1 can (14 oz) unsweetened coconut milk
- 3 tablespoons raw cacao powder
- 1 tablespoon maple syrup
- 1/8 teaspoon cardamom

Instructions:

1. Combine coconut cream and maple syrup in a bowl. Beat with a mixer until smooth and creamy.
2. Add cardamom and cacao and stir to combine, beat until smooth.
3. Cover and refrigerate before serving. Enjoy!

CHOCOLATE CUPCAKES

Cooking time: 20 minutes

Servings: 12

Ingredients:

- 1 cup whole wheat pastry flour
- 1 cup unsweetened almond or coconut milk
- ⅔ cup maple sugar
- 2 oz unsweetened vegan chocolate
- 1 teaspoon apple cider vinegar
- ¼ cup unsweetened applesauce
- 1 teaspoon vanilla extract
- ⅓ cup of cocoa powder
- ¾ teaspoon baking soda
- ½ teaspoon baking powder
- ¼ teaspoon salt

Instructions:

1. Preheat the oven to 350 F. Prepare a muffin pan and coat it with cooking spray.
2. Bring a pot of water to a boil over medium heat. Put the chocolate to a heatproof bowl and place it on top

of the pot. Stir until melted. Remove from heat and let cook for about 5 minutes.

3. Combine milk and vinegar in a bowl. Let rest for 5 minutes.

4. Add maple sugar, vanilla, applesauce, and chocolate and stir well to combine.

5. Mix flour, baking soda, baking powder, cocoa powder and salt in a separate bowl. Now add the flour mixture to the milk mixture and stir well until combined and smooth.

6. Pour the batter into the muffin pan and bake for 20 minutes.

7. Let cool before serving. Enjoy!

LEMON POPPY SEED SCONES

Cooking time: 10 minutes

Servings: 12

Ingredients:

- 1 3/4 cups all-purpose flour
- 1 tablespoon poppy seeds
- 1 lemon, zested
- 3/4 cup + 1 tablespoon soy milk
- 1 1/2 tablespoons sugar
- 1/4 cup coconut oil
- 1/2 tablespoon baking powder
- 1/2 teaspoon baking soda
- 1/2 teaspoon salt
  For the Glaze:
- 2 tablespoons soy milk, warm
- 1 tablespoon lemon juice
- 1 tablespoon lemon zest
- 3/4 cup icing sugar
- 1 tablespoon coconut oil, melted

Instructions:

1. Preheat the oven to 400 F. Prepare a baking sheet and line it with parchment paper.
2. Mix flour, poppy seeds, lemon zest, sugar, baking powder, baking soda and salt in a bowl.
3. Add coconut oil and mix well with a fork until crumbs are formed.
4. Add milk and stir well to combine. Transfer the dough onto the floured working surface and knead well for about 6-8 minutes. Roll out into 1 inch thick square.
5. Cut into triangles and place on the baking sheet. Bake for 10 minutes.
6. Mix all the glaze ingredients in a bowl. Drizzle over scones and serve. Enjoy!

CHOCOLATE CHIP COOKIES

Cooking time: 15 minutes

Servings: 20

Ingredients

- 2 cups plain flour
- 1 tablespoon soya milk
- 7 oz dairy-free margarine
- 7 oz vegan dark chocolate chips
- 1 cup soft light brown sugar
- Pinch of salt
- 3 ½ oz caster sugar
- ½ teaspoon bicarbonate of soda
- 1 teaspoon vanilla extract
- ½ teaspoon baking powder

Instructions

1. Take two baking trays lined with baking paper.
2. Take a bowl and combine vanilla extract, caster sugar, brown sugar and margarine. Then add pinch of salt, ½ teaspoon bicarbonate of soda, ½ teaspoon baking powder and flour; mix well until smooth.
3. Next, add 7 oz chocolate chips and 1 tablespoon soy milk; mix well again.

4. Scoop out dough, shape into balls, and place on the prepared baking trays. Make sure that there is enough space.

5. Bake until the cookies become golden for about 10-12 minutes. Take out from the oven and let them cool. Serve and enjoy!

BROWNIES

Cooking time: 30 minutes

Servings: 12

Ingredients

- 2 tablespoons maple syrup
- 3 ½ oz vegan chocolate chips (optional)
- 3 tablespoons ground flaxseed
- 2 tablespoons soya milk
- 200g vegan dark chocolate, chopped
- Pinch of salt
- 4 oz dairy-free margarine
- ½ teaspoon baking powder
- 1 cup caster sugar
- 1 cup plain flour
- 1 cup light muscovado sugar
- 1 teaspoon vanilla extract

Instructions

1. Grease a baking tin and line with parchment paper.
2. Take a bowl and mix 3 tablespoons flaxseeds along with cold water; whisk well; keep aside for 10-15 minutes.

3. Place a heatproof bowl in hot water pan and melt chocolate in it (water should not be in contact with the bowl). Add margarine when all of the chocolate is melted and turn off the heat. Margarine will melt in hot chocolate.

4. Add caster sugar, muscovado sugar, vanilla extract, and maple syrup into the chocolate; mix well until smooth.

5. Now take a bowl and add ½ teaspoon baking powder, a pinch of salt, and flour; mix until all the ingredients are incorporated.

6. Now transfer the batter to the baking tin; spread evenly; top with chocolate chips; bake in the preheated oven (375 F) for approximately 30 minutes.

7. Let the brownies cool; transfer to a big board and slice into squares.

NO-BAKE LEMON TARTS

Cooking time: 20 minutes + chilling time

Servings: 3 mini tarts

Ingredients

For the crust

- 2 tablespoons coconut oil melted
- 1 teaspoon lemon zest
- 1 cup coconut, shredded
- 2 tablespoons lemon juice
- ¾ cup raw cashews
- 2 tablespoons maple syrup

For the filling

- 4 tablespoons canned coconut milk
- 2 pinches of sea salt
- 1 cup raw cashews (soaked for at least 4 hours in cold water)
- 1 teaspoon vanilla extract
- ½ cup lemon juice
- 1 tablespoon lemon zest
- 5 tablespoons coconut oil
- 4 tablespoons maple syrup

Instructions

1. Grease a tart pan with coconut oil.

2. **For the crust**: Mix ¾ cup raw cashews and 1 cup shredded coconut in a blender/food processor and blend until the cashews are broken into smaller pieces. Now add 2 tablespoons maple syrup, 1 teaspoon lemon zest, 2 tablespoons coconut oil and 2 tablespoons lemon juice; blend until all the ingredients stick together.

3. Pour this mixture intothe prepared pan/s; keep it aside.

4. **For the filling:** Use the same blender and mix all the filling ingredients. Blend until a creamy mixture is obtained for 3-4 minutes. You can also add a little coconut oil to make the mixture smooth. After that, adjust lemon juice and maple syrup according to your taste.

5. Pour this smooth filling over the prepared crust. Make sure that the top must be smooth.

6. Put the pan into the refrigerator for 2-3 hours and then serve immediately.

PEANUT BUTTER CARAMEL RICE KRISPIES

Cooking time: 35 minutes

Servings: 9

Ingredients

- 5 tablespoons peanut butter
- 6 cups rice crisp cereal
- 3/4 cup brown rice syrup
- 1 teaspoon vanilla extract
- 4 tablespoons maple syrup

Peanut butter drizzle

- 1 teaspoon maple syrup
- 2 tablespoons creamy peanut butter
- 1–2 teaspoons water, if needed

Instructions

1. Line a square pan with wax paper/parchment paper.
2. Preheat 3/4 cup brown rice syrup and 4 tablespoons maple syrup in a pot over a medium-high flame; boil and cook for a minute with stirring. Turn off the heat.
3. Add 5 tablespoons peanut butter and 1 teaspoon vanilla extract in the pot and whisk until smooth.

4. Now add 6 cups rice crisp cereal and stir until well combined.
5. Spread this mixture in the pan evenly. Press lightly with a spatula; freeze for 10 minutes.
6. Take another bowl and combine 1 teaspoon maple syrup and 2 tablespoons peanut butter; microwave for 30 seconds. If needed, then add a teaspoon of water.
7. Take out the Krispies from the freezer; drizzle over peanut butter; again freeze until firm for at least 10-12 minutes.
8. Next, slice into cubes. Enjoy the chilled krispies!
9. Leftovers can be stored for 6-7 days in the fridge.

GUILT-FREE COCONUT VANILLA MACAROONS

Cooking time: 15 minutes

Servings: 1-2

Ingredients

- ¼ cup raw cane sugar
- 1 teaspoon vanilla extract
- 2 cups unsweetened shredded coconut
- 1 tablespoon almond flour
- 1 cup unsweetened almond milk
- 1 tablespoon coconut flour

Instructions

1. Place a parchment paper-lined baking dish into an oven and heat to 350°F.
2. Add sweetener and coconut milk to a saucepan; whisk together over medium heat.
3. Next, add flour, stirring continuously until all the clumps disappear.
4. Increase the heat to high and boil it until the mixture becomes thick for about 3-5 minutes.

5. Turn off the heat; add shredded coconut and vanilla and stir well.
6. Scoop 1 tablespoon mixture into the prepared baking dish; bake until golden brown for 15-17 minutes.
7. Cool to the room temperature and enjoy the meal!

GLUTEN-FREE BAKED CHOCOLATE DOUGHNUTS

Cooking time: 10 minutes

Servings: 6

Ingredients:

For the Doughnuts

- 2 pinches baking soda
- 1 teaspoon vanilla
- 1 tablespoon ground flax seeds
- 3 tablespoons coconut oil
- 3 tablespoons water
- 1/2 cup unsweetened non-dairy milk
- 3/4 cup gluten-free flour OR all-purpose flour
- 7 tablespoons coconut sugar
- 4 tablespoons unsweetened cocoa powder
- 1/4 teaspoon salt
- 1/2 teaspoon baking powder

For the Glaze

- 3/4 cup powdered sugar
- 1/8 teaspoon vanilla
- 2 tablespoons warm non-dairy milk

Instructions

1. Grease the doughnut pan.
2. For the flax egg: whisk flax seeds with water; keep aside until thickens.
3. Take a bowl and combine 2 pinches of baking soda, 7 tablespoons coconut sugar, 1/2 teaspoon baking powder, 4 tablespoons cocoa powder, 3/4 cup flour, and ¼ teaspoon salt.
4. Take another bowl and mix 3 tablespoons coconut oil, vanilla and milk along with flax mixture.
5. Combine wet and dry ingredients.
6. Transferthe mixture into the piping bag and pipe into the doughnut pan.
7. Bake in a preheated oven at 375°F for 10 minutes.Take out from the oven; leave for 5-10 minutes.
8. Now remove the doughnuts and place them on a cooling rack.
9. For the glaze: take a small bowl and mix all the Glaze ingredients in it.Dip the cooled doughnuts one by one into the glaze.
10. Place them into the cooling rack again so that the excess glaze will be drain off (place parchment paper under the rack).

PEANUT BUTTER FUDGE

Cooking time: 30 minutes

Servings: 21 (bars)

Ingredients

Fudge

- 1 teaspoon pure vanilla extract
- ¼ cup raw cane sugar
- 2 cups unsweetened coconut, finely shredded
- 3-5 tablespoon maple syrup (or any other sweetener of choice)
- 1 cup creamy peanut butter
- Coconut oil

Toppings (Optional)

- Coconut flakes
- Crushed peanuts

Instructions

1. Take a loaf pan (9x5-inch) and line with parchment paper; keep aside.
2. Add coconut milk in a food processor; blend for about 4 minutes until it becomes a creamy butter.

3. Add coconut oil and peanut butter; blend. Next, add maple syrup (add only 1 tablespoon at a time; it's up to you how much sweetness you need). The mixture can be extra thick if you add too much maple syrup. Add a bit of melted coconut oil if needed.

4. **Optional:** If you add vanilla and salt, then mix them again.

5. Pour this mixture to the prepared loaf pan and spread evenly. Top with Crushed peanuts and Coconut flakes if desired.

6. Freeze for about 15 to 20 minutes until firm. Slice the mixture into at least 21 even squares by using a hot knife. Enjoy it!

7. Leftovers can be stored in a freezer up to one month. Before serving, bring them to the room temperature.

TAHINI-STUFFED DATES

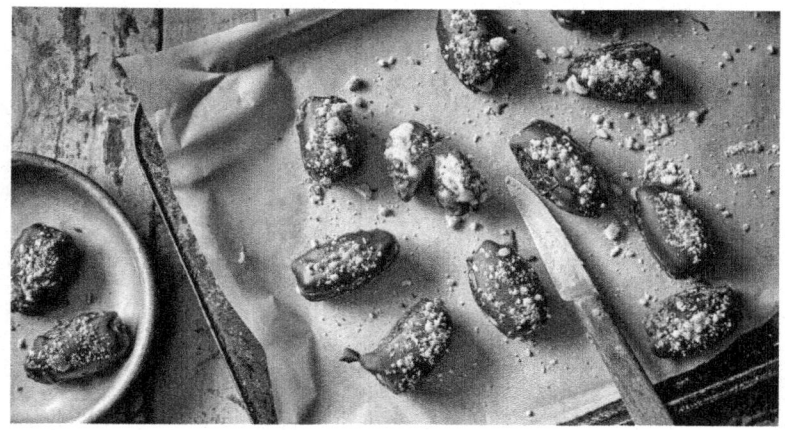

Cooking time: 5 minutes

Servings: 25 (stuffed dates)

Ingredients

Dates

- ¼ cup tahini (from raw or roasted sesame seeds)
- 2 tablespoons unsweetened desiccated coconut flake or sesame seeds
- 25 whole Medjool dates
- 1/8 teaspoon sea salt

Chocolate

- 2 tablespoons coconut oil
- 1 cup cacao or unsweetened cocoa powder

- 1 1/4 cups cocoa butter, finely chopped
- 2 tablespoons maple syrup

Instructions

1. Take a saucepan and add water up to 2 inches; boil and reduce the heat to low.
2. Now set a mixing bowl on top of the saucepan (remember, it should not be in contact with water).
3. Add coconut oil and cocoa butter to a mixing bowl; let them melt with occasional stirring for 3-4 minutes.
4. Turn off the heat once melted; add cocoa powder along with maple syrup; whisk well. Adjust sweetness according to your taste.
5. Refrigerate chocolate for 20-25 minutes. Remove pits from the dates and split them into two pieces.
6. Create small holes and stuff with tahini. Place dates onto the baking sheet, and freeze until chill.
7. Add dates one by one to the thick chocolate and coat it completely; remove excess chocolate.
8. Place them again on the baking sheet and sprinkle with salt, coconut/sesame seeds over it.
9. Enjoy the tahini-stuffed dates immediately.
10. Leftovers can be refrigerated for a week. Before serving, let them come to room temperature.

DARK CHOCOLATE TRUFFLES

Cooking time: 20 minutes + freezing time

Servings: 16 (truffles)

Ingredients

- ½ cup of coconut milk
- 4 tablespoons cacao powder/unsweetened cocoa
- 1/2 teaspoon vanilla extract (OPTIONAL)
- 1 1/4 cups vegan dark chocolate, finely chopped

Instructions

1. Take a bowl and add 1 1/4 cup finely chopped dark chocolate. Make sure that the chocolate is finely chopped so that it melts easily.
2. Add ½ cup coconut milk in a saucepan and heat over medium heat (alternatively, heat the milk in a microwave for just 25-30 seconds).
3. Next, pour hot coconut milk immediately over the chopped chocolate; cover the bowl loosely with a towel or a lid; leave for 5 minutes. Stir until the mixture becomes smooth, creamy, and melted.

4. After the mixture becomes completely smooth and melted, add 1/2 teaspoon vanilla extract and stir lightly.

5. Place this mixture into the refrigerator until it becomes completely solid, for 2-3 hours.

6. Now add cocoa powder to a separate dish for rolling.

7. Shape the mixture into balls and coat them with cocoa powder. Take the parchment-lined serving dish and place all the coated chocolate balls on it.

8. Again, if any chocolate remains soft then refrigerate it before scooping out. Enjoy the chocolate truffles, or you can also refrigerate them overnight.

9. Take out truffles from the refrigerator 10-15 minutes before serving.

TAHINI CHOCOLATE BANANA SOFT SERVE

Cooking time: 10 minutes

Servings: 2

Ingredients

- 3 tablespoons cacao powder
- 1/8 teaspoon sea salt (optional)
- 2 cups ripe frozen bananas, sliced
- 1 teaspoon vanilla extract (optional)
- 2 Tablespoons tahini (sesame seed paste or sub another nut/seed butter)
- 1-2 ripe pitted dates (optional)

Instructions

1. Add frozen bananas to a blender/food processor; blend until creamy.
2. Now add 3 tablespoons cacao powder, 2 tablespoons tahini (or seed butter), and pitted dates/maple syrup; blend again until combined.
3. Adjust flavors according to your taste. For more flavor, add a pinch of salt along with vanilla extract; mix well.

4. Transfer to a serving bowl and serve immediately. You can also freeze it for a few minutes before serving.

5. Leftovers can be freeze for a week. Before serving, let them come to room temperature.

THAI ICED TEA

Cooking time: 10 minutes

Servings: 4

Ingredients

- 4 tablespoons packed light muscovado sugar, coconut sugar or organic brown sugar

- 1-2 tablespoons dark rum per serving (optional)

- 4 cups of filtered water

- 1 14-ounce can light coconut milk (or other milk of your choice)

- 2 tablespoons *loose*-leaf black tea

- 1 teaspoon pure vanilla extract

- 4 tablespoons maple syrup/agave nectar

Instructions

1. Take a saucepan; add water, and bring to a boil.
2. Turn off the heat; leave for few minutes and add 2 tablespoons loose leaf black tea, stir well. Again leave for 5-10 minutes.

3. Strain the tea. Add 4 tablespoons maple syrup, 1 teaspoon pure vanilla extract, and 4 tablespoons muscovado sugar. Whisk until sugar dissolves. You can adjust sweetness according to your taste; refrigerate for 2-3 hours.
4. Pour chilled tea into the serving glasses on top of ice cubes.
5. Fill the glass until 3/4 full; pour coconut milk over it and stir. To make a creamy cocktail, add 1-2 tablespoons dark rum per glass.

CHAI TEA LATTES

Cooking time: 15 minutes

Servings: 2 lattes

Ingredients

Chai Latte

- 2 cups Water
- Coconut whip cream, optional
- 1-2 tablespoons chai spice mix
- 2 tablespoons maple syrup
- 2 black tea bags
- 1 cup oat milk (or any other plant milk)

Chai Spice Mix

- 1.5 teaspoon ground ginger
- pinch of nutmeg
- 1 tablespoon ground cinnamon
- 1 teaspoon allspice
- 2 teaspoon ground cardamom

Instructions

1. Take a saucepan and add water along with chai spice mix; boil it. Once boiled, turn the heat off; leave for a

few minutes. Now add 2 tablespoons maple syrup and 2 black tea bags and boil again; again turn the heat off and leave for a few minutes.

2. Remove the teabags, pour this mixture into two cups.

3. Heat oat milk and add into the cups; mix well. Sprinkle with cinnamon and top with coconut whip.

LEMON TULSI TEA

Cooking time: 5 minutes

Servings: 1

Ingredients

- 8 oz water, boiling
- 1 bag tulsi tea
- 1 tablespoon maple syrup or 1 teaspoon sugar
- 1 tablespoon lemon juice

Instructions

1. Add maple syrup and lemon juice to a cup and pour the boiling water on top.
2. Add the teabag and leave it for 5 minutes.
3. Remove the bag and serve tea.

PEACH ICED TEA

Cooking time: 15 minutes

Servings: 2

Ingredients

- 1 ½ peach, sliced
- ½ cup of sugar
- 1-2 tea bags
- ½ cup of water

Instructions

1. Add peaches and sugar to a pan, cover with water. Simmer for 5 minutes.
2. Mash the peaches and cook over low heat for 10 minutes more.
3. Remove from heat; let stand for 30 minutes.
4. Sieve the mixture. Make the black tea (4 cups) and let cool.
5. Add peach mixture and tea to the glasses over ice. Serve.

ROOIBOS AND PEAR TEA

Cooking time: 5 minutes

Servings: 2

Ingredients

- 1 pear, sliced
- 2 teaspoons black tea leaves
- ½ cinnamon stick

Instructions

1. Add pears to a pan, cover with water. Simmer for 5 minutes.
2. Add tea leaves and let rest for 2-3 minutes. Sieve the tea and add the cinnamon stick. Serve.

TURMERIC TEA

Cooking time: 5 minutes

Servings: 2

Ingredients

- 1 orange, zested
- 1 tablespoon fresh ginger, minced
- 3 teaspoons turmeric
- Agave syrup
- Lemon slices

Instructions

1. Bring 2 cups water to a boil.
2. Add turmeric, orange zest and ginger to cups and pour the water on top. Stir to combine.
3. Serve with agave syrup and lemon slices.

GREEN TEA WITH GRAPEFRUIT

Cooking time: 5 minutes

Servings: 2

Ingredients

- ¼ grapefruit, sliced
- 2 teaspoons tea leaves
- A sprig rosemary
- Agave syrup, to taste

Instructions

1. Bring 2 cups water to a boil.
2. Add tea and let rest for 2-3 minutes. Add grapefruit and rosemary to a cup and pour the tea on top.
3. Serve with agave syrup to taste.

MINT TEA

Cooking time: 5 minutes

Servings: 2

Ingredients

- A handful of mint leaves
- Agave syrup, to taste
- Water

Instructions

1. Bring 2 cups water to a boil.
2. Add mint leaves and let it infuse for 5 minutes.
3. Serve with agave syrup to taste.

SUNSHINE SMOOTHIE

Prep time: 5 minutes

Servings: 3

Ingredients

- 2 bananas, sliced into chunks
- 1 lime, juiced
- 2 cups carrot juice, chilled
- 1 tablespoon cashew nuts
- 7 oz pineapple, fresh or canned
- A small piece of ginger, peeled

Instructions

1. Add all smoothie ingredients to a blender or a food processor.
2. Blitz until smooth and combined.
3. Pour into chilled glasses and serve. Enjoy!

YOUTHFUL GREEN SMOOTHIE

Prep time: 5 minutes

Servings: 4

Ingredients

- 1/2 cucumber
- 1 teaspoon fresh ginger, grated
- 2 handfuls kale or power greens mix
- ice
- 2 oz baby spinach
- 1 banana
- 2 cups apple juice
- 1/2 lemon, squeezed

Instructions

1. Add all smoothie ingredients to a blender or a food processor.
2. Blitz until smooth and combined.
3. Pour into chilled glasses and serve. Enjoy!

ORANGE CARDAMOM BEET SMOOTHIE

Prep time: 10 minutes

Servings: 1-2

Ingredients

- 2 pinches of ground cardamom
- 1-inch piece of fresh ginger, peeled
- 1 small beet, peeled
- 1 cup orange juice
- 1 large frozen banana

Instructions

1. Add all smoothie ingredients to a blender or a food processor.
2. Blitz until smooth and combined.
3. Pour into chilled glasses and serve. Enjoy!

PEACHY MANGO SMOOTHIE

Prep time: 5 minutes

Servings: 4

Ingredients

- 1 banana
- 1/4 teaspoon ginger
- 7 oz peach chunks
- 2 pinches of turmeric
- 5 oz mangoes
- 1 cup of orange juice

Instructions

1. Add all smoothie ingredients to a blender or a food processor.
2. Blitz until smooth and combined.
3. Pour into chilled glasses and serve. Enjoy!

GINGER AND SPINACH GREEN SMOOTHIE

Prep time: 5 minutes

Servings: 2

Ingredients

- ice cubes
- 1/3 cucumber, cut into 2.5 cm chunks
- 1 cup oforange juice
- 1-2 tablespoons fresh ginger, minced
- 1 cup of coconut yogurt
- 1 handful fresh baby spinach
- 7 oz frozen mango chunks

Instructions

1. Add all smoothie ingredients to a blender or a food processor.
2. Blitz until smooth and combined.
3. Pour into chilled glasses and serve. Enjoy!

OIL-FREE BALSAMIC DRESSING

Prep time: 2 minutes

Servings: 2

Ingredients

- ¼ teaspoon dried basil
- 2 teaspoons balsamic vinegar
- 1 teaspoon Dijon mustard
- 1 teaspoon nutritional yeast
- 2 teaspoons water
- Sea salt, pepper, to taste

Instructions

1. Mix all sauce ingredients in a bowl.
2. Stir well to combine. Refrigerate before serving.

CREAMY RED PEPPER CORIANDER SAUCE

Prep time: 15 minutes

Servings: 2-4

Ingredients

- 1 extra package firm silken tofu, drained
- 2 red bell peppers, roasted and seeded
- ¼ cup cilantro, chopped
- 3 garlic cloves, peeled and chopped
- 1 lime, zested and juiced
- 1 teaspoon salt
- ½ teaspoon crushed red pepper

Instructions

1. Mix all sauce ingredients in a blender or a food processor. Blitz well to combine.
2. Refrigerate before serving.

NACHO CHEESE SAUCE

Prep time: 5 minutes

Servings: 2

Ingredients

- 1 cup non-dairy yogurt
- 3 tablespoons flour
- 1 1/4 cups vegetable broth
- 1/4 teaspoon garlic salt
- 1/2 teaspoon cumin
- 1 teaspoon chili powder
- 1/4 teaspoon paprika
- 1/4 teaspoon salt
- A pinch cayenne

Instructions

1. Add broth to a pan and bring to a boil.
2. Mix yogurt and flour in a bowl. Reduce the heat to low and add the flour mixture to the broth. Stir well to combine.
3. Add all the spices and bring to a simmer. Let cool and serve.

RANCH DRESSING

Prep time: 15 minutes

Servings: 8-10

Ingredients

- 1/2 cup soy milk
- 1 cup vegan mayonnaise
- 1 tablespoon dill, chopped
- 2 teaspoons parsley, chopped
- 1/2 teaspoon garlic powder
- 1/2 teaspoon onion powder
- 1/4 teaspoon black pepper

Instructions

1. Mix all sauce ingredients in a bowl.
2. Stir well to combine. Refrigerate before serving.

BARBECUE TAHINI SAUCE

Prep time: 10 minutes

Servings: 8-10

Ingredients

- ¼ - ½ cup of water
- 6 tablespoons tahini
- 10 teaspoons tomato paste
- 2 teaspoons maple syrup
- 3 teaspoons apple cider vinegar
- 3 teaspoons molasses
- 1/4 teaspoon liquid smoke
- 1/8 teaspoon chili powder
- 3/4 teaspoon garlic powder
- sea salt , to taste

Instructions

1. Mix all sauce ingredients in a blender or a food processor. Blitz well to combine.
2. Refrigerate before serving.

WHOLE ROASTED CAULIFLOWER WITH TAHINI SAUCE

Cooking time: 75 minutes

Servings: 4

Ingredients

- ½ teaspoon salt
- 1 cup of water
- 1 whole cauliflower
- 1 tablespoon zaatar spice (or a combination of cumin, coriander, and optional sumac)
- 2 tablespoons olive oil

    For Garnishing:

- Parsley, dill and or mint
- Aleppo chili flakes
- Tahini sauce

Instructions

1. Trim and slice the cauliflower from the bottom; place them in an ovenproof skillet.
2. Drizzle olive oil over it; sprinkle with zaatar spice and salt.

3. Take a cup of water and pour in the bottom of the pan; cover the pan with foil tightly.

4. Place the pan into the preheated oven at 425F and bake for 50-55 minutes.

5. Remove the foil, drizzle with little olive oil, and again bake until it becomes completely golden for 30 minutes.

6. Take out from the oven; sprinkle with fresh herbs and aleppo chili flakes; drizzle with the prepared sauce.

7. Cut into wedges like a cake and serve with tahini sauce. Enjoy the meal!

MUSHROOM PASTA WITH ROASTED SUNCHOKES

Cooking time: 20 minutes

Servings: 3-4

Ingredients

- 8 oz dry pasta (fettuccine, tagliatelle, linguine, spaghetti)
- 2 teaspoon olive oil
- 8 ounces sunchokes
- 8 ounces mushrooms, sliced
- 2 teaspoons olive oil
- Salt, to taste
- Pepper, to taste
- Artichoke Sauce:
- 10 fresh sage leaves
- 1 jar artichoke hearts or use frozen
- ½ teaspoon cracked pepper
- ½ cup of water
- ½ teaspoon salt
- ¼ cup olive oil
- 2 garlic cloves
- Lemon juice, to taste
- For Garnishing: (Optional)

- Pecorino, grated
- Truffle oil

Instructions

1. Wash the sunchokes and pat dry; quarter them; toss with olive oil in a bowl along with pepper and salt; place on a baking sheet lined with parchment paper and roast in the preheated oven at 400 F until tender for about 20 minutes.

2. Take a big pot and add water and salt to it; bring to a boil — Cook pasta as per the package directions.

3. Take a large skillet and fry mushrooms in a little olive oil over medium heat; sprinkle pepper and salt over it; keep aside.

4. **For Artichoke Sauce**: Add drained artichoke hearts into a blender/food processor; add all the Artichoke Sauce ingredients. Blitz until smooth and creamy.

5. Now add cooked pasta into the mushrooms; toss them with prepared artichoke sauce; heat it while stirring gently.

6. Add more salt if needed.Next, add roasted sunchokes; mix well.

7. Drizzle with truffle oil. You can also sprinkle with chili flakes.

BERRY BANANA SMOOTHIE BOWL

Cooking time: 10 minutes

Servings: 1

Ingredients

- 1 cup frozen pineapple
- 2 tablespoons unsweetened coconut flakes
- 1/2 cup unsweetened almond milk
- 1/4 cup blackberries
- 1 cup baby spinach leaves
- 10 salted almonds, crushed
- 2 tablespoons chia seeds
- 1 banana, sliced
- 1 cup frozen blueberries
- 1/2 cup carrots, chopped

Instructions

1. Add all the smoothie ingredients (except coconut flakes, blackberries, and crushed almonds) to a high speed blender.

2. Blitz to combine, until smooth and creamy.

3. Pour into a bowl and serve with the remaining ingredients.

SWEET POTATO DHAL

Cooking time: 50 minutes

Servings: 2-3

Ingredients

For the Spices:

- 1 tablespoon ginger, grated
- 1 teaspoon ground turmeric
- 1 tablespoon Indian curry powder

For the Dhal:

- 2 garlic cloves, crushed
- 1 cup spinach leaves
- 1 cup red lentils (soaked in water overnight)
- 1 medium red chili chopped (if you need spicy)
- 2 cups sweet potato, chopped
- 1 lime juice
- 2 cups vegetable broth
- 1 large onion
- 1 cup of organic coconut milk
- 1 tablespoon coconut oil

For the Topping:

- Lime juice
- Fresh coriander

Instructions

1. Preheat oil in a pot over medium-high heat; sauté garlic and onion along with spices for 2-3 minutes.
2. Rinse lentils with water; place in the pot along with all the leftover ingredients (except spinach); simmer until the potato becomes soft for about 35-40 minutes.
3. Turn off the heat.Add spinach and mash potato by using a wooden spoon to get the dhal; leave for 10-15 minutes.
4. Top with coriander and lime juice and serve with rice.

SIMPLE BAKED SHEET-PAN RATATOUILLE

Cooking time: 60 minutes

Servings: 4-6

Ingredients

- 1 onion

- Splash of balsamic vinegar

- 3 Japanese eggplants

- Salt, to taste

- Pepper, to taste

- 1 red or yellow bell pepper

- Olive oil, for drizzling

- 2 medium tomatoes

- 2–3 tablespoon fresh herbs (rosemary or thyme or combination of both)

- 2 zucchini

- 12–14 garlic cloves

Optional Garnishes:

- Italian parsley
- Fresh basil
- Capers
- Chili flakes
- Olive oil

Easy Creamy Polenta

- 1 tablespoon olive oil/butter
- Salt, to taste
- Pepper, to taste
- 1 cup of cornmeal
- ½ cup grated vegan cheese
- 4 ½ cups water or stock

Instructions

1. Place the parchment-lined pan into the preheated oven to 400 F. Peel eggplant with a peeler.Slice eggplant, tomatoes, bell pepper, zucchini and onion.

2. Spread all the vegetables in a single layer onto the prepared pan. Add herbs and peeled garlic cloves.

3. Drizzle olive oil over it; sprinkle with pepper and salt. Bake for 20 minutes; mix well; roast again for 20 minutes. Reduce the heat to 300F and roast again for about 15-20 minutes.

4. Adjust salt; drizzle vinegar over it.

5. If you want to serve your dish with Creamy Polenta, then follow these steps: take a medium pot and add 4 ½ cups water or stock; boil it. Add polenta slowly into the pot while vigorous whisking; cover it; reduce the heat and cook for 15-17 minutes.

6. Add ½ cup grated cheese, 1 tablespoon butter, pepper, and salt.

7. Pour into the bowls; top with warm Ratatouille; sprinkle with parsley/basil.

RAW APPLE PIE

Cooking time: 10 minutes

Servings: 4

Ingredients

- 1 1/2 teaspoons cinnamon

- 1 cup walnuts, chopped

- 4 apples, peeled and chopped

- 1 cup large dates, pitted and chopped

- 2 tablespoons lemon juice

Instructions

1. Mix all the ingredients (except walnuts) together in a bowl; leave for 30 minutes.
2. Top with chopped walnuts.Enjoy!

QUICK MUSHROOM AND LIME SALAD

Cooking time: 10 minutes

Servings: 2

Ingredients

- 1 tablespoon olive oil

- 8 green onions, thinly sliced

- 1/3 cup toasted peanuts

- 1 lime, juiced

- 1 cup cilantro, basil, mint, chopped

- 1/2 serrano, minced

- 1 lb mixed mushrooms, sliced into 1/4-inch thick pieces

- 1 tablespoon soy sauce

For Serving:

- Sprouts

- Micro greens

Instructions

1. Take a bowl and combine 8 thinly sliced green onions, 1 tablespoon soy sauce and ½ minced Serrano; keep aside.

2. Preheat olive oil in skillet over medium heat; add mushroom and sprinkle salt over it. Cook until mushrooms are brown for 5-6 minutes; once golden, then turn off the heat.

3. Transfer the golden mushrooms into the prepared scallion mixture; toss gently. Add toasted peanuts and herbs; drizzle soy sauce, if desired.

4. Top with sprouts and microgreens.

LENTIL BURGER WITH MUSTARD SAUCE

Cooking time: 30 minutes

Servings: 2-3

Ingredients

For the Mustard Sauce:

- 3 tablespoons yellow mustard

- A pinch of curry (optional)

- ¼ cup maple syrup

For the Lentil Burger Patties:

- 1/2 cup walnuts, crushed

- 1 cup uncooked lentils

- 2 tablespoons mustard sauce (optional)

- 5 tablespoons raisins

- 1 cup gluten-free bread crumbs

- Salt, to taste

For Toppings:

- Lettuce

- Roasted onions

- Tomato

Instructions

1. **Mustard Sauce:** Take a small bowl and mix ¼ cup maple syrup, 3 tablespoons yellow mustard, and a pinch of curry (optional).
2. **Lentil Burger Patties:** Cook lentils as per instructions are given on the packet and transfer it to a blender; add 1/2 cup walnuts and 5 tablespoons raisins; blend until chunky.
3. Take another bowl; add the lentil mixture along with bread crumbs; leave for 10 minutes.
4. Shape the mixture into patties.You can fry them in a pan (with little oil), or you can also bake them in the oven (at 390°F).
5. **Burger:** Now, take your favorite toppings for the burger and serve on the vegan buns.

30 DAYS MEAL PLAN

Day 1

BreakfastApple Buckwheat Pancakes With Coconut Caramel Apples

Lunch Roasted Vegetable Soup with Couscous

DinnerItalian Rice Noodles

SnackPotato Chips

Day 2

BreakfastQuick Vegan Breakfast Burritos

Lunch Fennel Asparagus Salad

DinnerMaple Glazed Tofu

DessertTahini Chocolate Banana Soft Serve

Day 3

BreakfastChickpea Omelette

Lunch Spicy Roasted Parsnip Soup

DinnerSpaghetti with Kale

SnackCrackers with Edamame Hummus

Day 4

Breakfast Gingerbread Waffles

Lunch Farro Tabbouleh Salad

Dinner Lasagne (Vegan version)

DessertDark ChocolateTruffles

Day 5

Breakfast Jelly-Filled Muffins

Lunch Minty Pea and Potato Soup

Dinner Spanish Vegan Paella

SnackPeanut Butter Jelly Apple Nachos

Day 6

Breakfast Toast with Refried Beans and Avocado

Lunch Cream of Mushroom Soup

Dinner Artichoke Mushroom Pizza

DessertTahini-Stuffed Dates

Day 7

Breakfast Sun-dried Tomato, Mushroom, and Spinach Tofu Quiche

Lunch Beetroot and Lentil Tabbouleh

Dinner Tomato Chili Bean

SnackFried Cinnamon Bananas

Day 8

Breakfast Vegan Breakfast Sandwich

Lunch Creamy Cauliflower Horseradish Soup

Dinner Sweet Potato Squash with Rice

DessertPeanut Butter Fudge

Day 9

Breakfast Warm and Nutty Cinnamon Quinoa

Lunch No-Cook Chickpea Salad

Dinner Curry Beans

SnackMaple Almond Popcorn

Day 10

Breakfast Canal House Lentils

Lunch Silky Cauliflower Soup

Dinner Fried Tofu and Edamame

DessertGluten-Free Baked Chocolate Doughnuts

Day 11

Breakfast Hot Chocolate Banana-Nut Oatmeal

Lunch Roasted Beets, Plum, and Pecan Salad

Dinner Chili Spaghetti

SnackTurmeric Snack Balls

Day 12

Breakfast Peanut Butter Banana Bread Granola

Lunch Roasted Red Pepper Tomato Soup

Dinner French Stewed Vegetable (Ratatouille)

DessertGuilt-Free Coconut Vanilla Macaroons

Day 13

Breakfast Broccoli and Quinoa Breakfast Patties

Lunch Avocado Panzanella

Dinner Spinach Puree and Sautéed Chickpea

SnackHerbed Fingerling Potatoes

Day 14

Breakfast Salted Caramel Apple Breakfast Bars

Lunch Glowing Carrot Ginger Soup

Dinner Pasta with Beans

DessertPeanut Butter Caramel Rice Krispies

Day 15

Breakfast Sweet Potato Breakfast Bowl

Lunch Butter Bean, Cucumber and Radish Salad

Dinner Vegan Enchiladas

SnackGrilled Portobello Mushrooms

Day 16

Breakfast Grits Bowl with Avocado and Baked Tofu Strips

Lunch Quinoa Black Bean Pumpkin Soup

Dinner Stuffed Peppers

DessertNo-Bake Lemon Tarts

Day 17

Breakfast Greek Chickpeas on Toast

Lunch Heirloom Tomato Salad

Dinner Fried Pad Thai Rice Noodles

SnackJordanian Spiced Roasted Chickpeas

Day 18

BreakfastBreakfast Hash

Lunch Healing Thai Butternut Squash Lentil Soup

Dinner Juicy Sautéed Mushrooms and Corn

DessertBrownies

Day 19

Breakfast Spinach Artichoke Quiche

Lunch Spiralized Zucchini and Carrot Salad

Dinner Saffron Quinoa with Pistachios

SnackSpicy French Fries

Day 20

Breakfast Fried Tofu

Lunch Winter Moroccan Sweet Potato Lentil Soup

Dinner Sautéed Cabbage

DessertChocolate Chip Cookies

Day 21

Breakfast Turmeric Tofu

Lunch Kale Power Salad with Lemon Tahini Dressing

Dinner Fried Rice

SnackCrusted Asparagus Spears

Day 22

Breakfast Deli-Style Vegan Cream Cheese Bowls

Lunch Spring Vegetable Quinoa Minestrone

Dinner Zucchini Balls with Pasta

DessertLemon Poppy Seed Scones

Day 23

Breakfast Cardamom and Peach Quinoa Porridge

Lunch Cranberry Cilantro Quinoa Salad

DinnerSloppy Joes

SnackBuffalo Cauliflower Bites

Day 24

Breakfast Three-Grain Porridge

Lunch Power Lentil Soup

DinnerRisotto

DessertChocolate Cupcakes

Day 25

BreakfastBreakfast Fry-Up

Lunch Sweet Potato Salad

DinnerMilky Cauliflower Pasta Mushroom Pasta with Roasted Sunchokes

SnackVegan 'Bacon' Strips

Day 26

Breakfast Peanut Butter Banana Bread Granola

Lunch Roasted Vegetable Soup with Couscous

DinnerSweet Potato Dhal

DessertCoconut Chocolate Mousse

Day 27

Breakfast Canal House Lentils

Lunch Fennel Asparagus Salad

DinnerSimple Baked Sheet-Pan Ratatouille

SnackFudgy Double Chocolate Apple Muffins

Day 28

Breakfast Gingerbread Waffles

Lunch Spicy Roasted Parsnip Soup

DinnerLentil Burger with Mustard Sauce

DessertLemon-Oatmeal Cookies

Day 29

Breakfast Apple Buckwheat Pancakes With Coconut Caramel Apples

Lunch Farro Tabbouleh Salad

DinnerItalian Rice Noodles

SnackSalted Caramel Apple Bars

Day 30

Breakfast Quick Vegan Breakfast Burritos

Lunch Minty Pea and Potato Soup

DinnerMaple Glazed Tofu

DessertLemon Cheesecake

CONCLUSION

This book can be your first guide for Plant-Based Diet if you just started your journey. Or it can help you with the recipe choice if you are already following the diet.

The Plant-Based and Alkaline diet is suitable for anyone who wants to improve the quality of everyday life. These diets can help to reduce the risk of heart disease, type 2 diabetes, cancer, premature death, Alzheimer's disease, various cancers, avoid side effects linked to the antibiotics and hormones used in modern animal agriculture, lower body weight and body mass index (BMI).

Usually, people decide to go vegan due to one or several reasons. People might switch to veganism due to their ethical reasons, as they believe all live creatures have a right to live, be free, and fairly treated. You can find your reasons.

There are many sources of healthy nutrients in vegan products. So you don't have to worry about getting enough vitamins to your body. This book will help you to make a healthy vegan Meal Plan for the whole family and spend less time in the kitchen.

Remember that Veganism is not only about the diet, but about changing your lifestyle to a more healthy and balanced one.

And this book will help you with this. You can choose the recipe you like from a variety of options:

- Breakfast recipes

- Bread and Biscuits

- Salads and Soups

- Main dishes

- Smoothies and Teas

- Sauces and condiments

- Desserts

- Snacks

- Whole Food recipes

DISCLAIMER

The information contained in this eBook is offered for informational purposes solely, and it is geared towards providing exact and reliable information in regards to the topic and issue covered. The author and the publisher does not warrant that the information contained in this e-book is fully complete and shall not be responsible for any errors or omissions.

The author and publisher shall have neither liability nor responsibility to any person or entity concerning any reparation, damages, or monetary loss caused or alleged to be caused directly or indirectly by this e-book. Therefore, this eBook should be used as a guide - not as the ultimate source.

The publication is sold with the idea that the publisher is not required to render accounting, officially permitted, or otherwise, qualified services. If advice is necessary, legal or professional, a practiced individual in the profession should be ordered.

In no way is it legal to reproduce, duplicate, or transmit any part of this document in either electronic means or printed format. Recording of this publication is strictly prohibited, and any storage of this document is not allowed unless with written permission from the publisher. All rights reserved.

Made in the USA
Monee, IL
11 December 2019